Get Healthy
...for Heaven's Sake

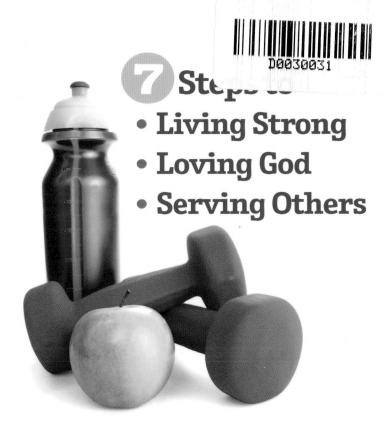

7 Steps to
- **Living Strong**
- **Loving God**
- **Serving Others**

LISA MORRONE, P.T.

Author of *Diabetes: Are You at Risk?*

Help for Healthy Living—
Praise for Other Books by Lisa Morrone, P.T.

Overcoming Overeating:

"A practical, sustainable, and results-oriented approach that will guide you to permanent mind change…*Overcoming Overeating* provides both the why and the how toward becoming the new, healthy you."

—J. RON EAKER, MD
physician and author of *Fat-Proof Your Family*

"A comprehensive remedy for weight loss. Lisa rightly views weight problems as having their origin in not just physical, but also mental, emotional, and spiritual arenas… An invaluable resource to the countless people struggling in this area of their life."

—DAVID HAWKINS, PhD
psychologist and author of
When Pleasing Others Is Hurting You

Overcoming Headaches and Migraines:

"A gift to headache sufferers and those in the health professions who are committed to helping them."

—HOWARD MAKOFSKY, PT, DHSc, OCS
head pain expert

"Lisa Morrone's extensive preparation, research, and years of experience are reflected in the safe and clinically proven techniques she recommends. A must-read for primary and specialty providers…and of course, anyone who suffers from headaches."

—WILLIAM ROBERT SPENCER, MD, FAAP
ear, nose, and throat specialist

Overcoming Back and Neck Pain:

"The treatments recommended are practical, well described, and well illustrated…An invaluable resource."

—JOHN LABIAK, MD
orthopaedist and spinal surgeon

"A very practical approach to the key things patients really need to know. I recommend it to all sufferers from spine problems...I appreciate Lisa's treatment of every person as someone who has not only a body and mind, but a spirit as well."

—Kent Keyser, MS, PT, OCS, COMT, ATC, FFCFMT, FAAOMPT
practicing and teaching physical therapist

Diabetes:

"I love this book because it takes you on a journey through diabetes and then gives you a light at the end of the tunnel, teaching how to prevent type 2 diabetes and how to reverse the pre-diabetic state and metabolic syndrome. Should be read by everyone interested in living a full and healthy life."

—Mariano Castro-Magana, MD
director, pediatric endocrinology and metabolism,
Winthrop Hospital, Mineola, New York

Get Healthy
...for Heaven's Sake

LISA MORRONE, P.T.

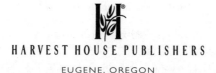

HARVEST HOUSE PUBLISHERS

EUGENE, OREGON

Cover by Koechel Peterson & Associates, Inc., Minneapolis, Minnesota

Cover photo © iStockphoto / Thinkstock; interior photos and graphics and
back-cover author photo © Peter Morrone

Illustrations by Rose C. Miller

Lisa Morrone is published in association with William K. Jensen Literary Agency, 119 Bampton Court, Eugene, Oregon 97404.

Readers are advised to consult with their physician or other professional practitioner before implementing any suggestions that follow. This book is not intended to take the place of sound professional advice, medical or otherwise. Neither the author nor the publisher assumes any liability for possible adverse consequences as a result of the information contained herein.

GET HEALTHY, FOR HEAVEN'S SAKE
Copyright © 2011 by Lisa Morrone, P.T.
Published by Harvest House Publishers
Eugene, Oregon 97402
www.harvesthousepublishers.com

Library of Congress Cataloging-in-Publication Data
    Morrone, Lisa, 1967-
    Get healthy, for heaven's sake / Lisa Morrone.
        p. cm.
    Includes bibliographical references.
    ISBN 978-0-7369-2704-8 (pbk.)
    1. Health. 2. Health—Religious aspects—Christianity. I. Title.
    RA776.5.M635 2011
    613—dc22

                                            2010021577

Printed in the United States of America

11 12 13 14 15 16 17 18 19 / VP-SK / 10 9 8 7 6 5 4 3 2 1

This book is dedicated to you—yes, you, its reader. Each day as I sat down to write I thought of you and have prayed for just the right words to encourage you along your journey toward better health and more vibrant living. May you find hope, healing, and health on each page!

ACKNOWLEDGMENTS

This book is the direct result of Your "new vocational call" on my life back in 2006, Lord Jesus. Without Your Holy Spirit's prompting, this book and all the others I've written would not have come to be. I am humbled by the tens of thousands who have read and been helped by my words of instruction and healing. May Your ministry continue through me, and may I always be willing to respond in obedience when You call my name—the first time.

Contents

PART 1

GOD'S PLANS FOR YOUR GOOD HEALTH

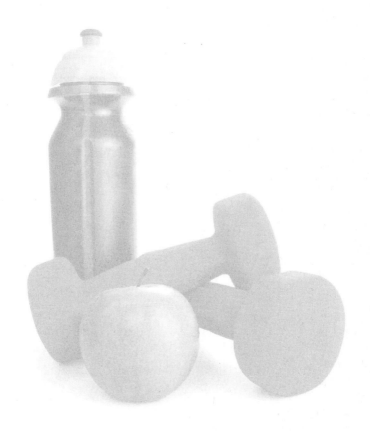

1

Investing in Your Future
Making the Most of God's Gift of Life

Let this be written for a future generation, that a
people not yet created may praise the LORD.

PSALM 102:18

I t was the summer before I was to begin the fifth grade. On the very
same day the world lost Elvis, the king of rock 'n' roll, I lost my "second mother," my Aunt Catherine, to breast cancer. She was only
52. And though that loss was devastating for me, God was true to His
promise "to make all things work together for good, for those who love
Him and are called according to His purpose." Within the very hour of
my aunt's death, my uncle—fresh in his grief—drew me into his arms
and said, "Lisa, I want you to promise me that you will always take care
of your body. Make sure you keep yourself healthy."

At ten years old, I stood there stunned. Up to that point I had
always assumed that sickness or disease was something that just "happened" to people. It had never occurred to me that humans had the
power to positively (or negatively) influence their future health. Having watched my aunt suffer terribly throughout my childhood, and
having seen how her longing to play a vital role in the Christian community went unrealized, I determined that, as far as it depended on
me, I would walk a different road and make the necessary investments
to ensure that I had a healthy future.

Investments of any kind are best realized when we use some fore-
thought. As a rule of thumb, the sooner you begin investing, the better

off you are in the future. For example, when it comes to finances, if you're like me, you may feel frustrated with yourself for not having begun saving years earlier. Sooner or later it dawns on us that in order to achieve maximal return on our investments, we need to take advantage of the principle of compounding interest. In giving advice to those who've yet to begin investing, financial gurus always recommend that *now* is the best time to begin.

The same "compounding principle" holds true of your health. In order to achieve maximum returns, you must take care to invest in the wellness of your body *today* if you expect to reap great rewards tomorrow, next year, and in the years to come. The sooner you start, the more health you can have in the future, and the less disease and disability you will have to deal with.

Healthful changes implemented today will yield fabulous returns in this life—both short-term and long-term. For example, getting a good night's sleep tonight will not only give you a better outlook tomorrow, but it will also help to prevent aging, improve brain function, and assist you in losing those stubborn extra pounds. Becoming proactive in your own health care is the very best way to preserve and protect your life. If you work at reversing the effects of neglect or abuse and then seek to maintain your physical well-being, you will be poised to do far more for the kingdom of God.

Investing in your wellness will yield great dividends for all eternity. One of God's most precious blessings to us is the physical body we each have been given. The Bible tells us that we are the only part of God's creation that was made in His image. Integral to His creation are our physical bodies, with which we worship and bring glory to Him through performing good works—or as my Southern girlfriends would say, "being Jesus with skin on." With our bodies we serve the needs of other Christians and bring the gospel message to the unsaved. We've been created to bring God glory by using our physical strength.

Switching Plans

Before the introduction of sin into the world, the Bible tells us that these bodies of ours did not see decay. Amazing, huh? No wrinkle creams or walking canes were needed; no reading glasses or gray hair to deal with. As we age, however, we become all too aware that we aren't the same today as we were last year—or the year before, for that matter. Disease and decay are part of Satan's plan to destroy our bodies, one of God's most precious creations. The systematic breakdown of a believer's body effectively, and progressively, reduces his or her usefulness in serving Christ on this earth.

And you know what? From a strategic point of view, Satan has done well for himself. Today, the lifestyles of many of us have left us vulnerable to sickness and disability. At times we are even playing for the wrong side—helping Satan with his own game plan for our early demise. We're abusing our bodies by overeating, not getting enough sleep, or by feeding our brains a steady diet of health-depleting thoughts and food choices.

Well, this book presents a different plan, and it brings an entirely different outlook for your future! There is much that can be done to resist, reverse, and reconstruct the aging process. Getting older is irreversible—a result of the original sin—but the *way* in which we age, and the *speed* at which we deteriorate, are very much under our control. Because there's a battle raging, a spiritual one, to participate fully we need to be ready, willing, and most important…*able*. Has the lifestyle you've chosen caused you to lay down your weapon of warfare (your physical body) on the couch to rest or on a doctor's exam table? Isn't it time to get up? You and I belong on the battlefield. It's why we were created!

The Essential Components of Wellness

From the knowledge I've gained during my 20-plus years of patient care in the medical field (and my 40-some years of personal and spiritual life experience as a born-again believer), I see *six essential components of wellness* a person needs to pursue, restore, and maintain optimal physical health.

- The first area to address is *sleep*—that is, the lack of it.
  Sleep is not simply downtime; it is repair and rejuvenation

time for your body and your brain. Seventy-four percent
of people report regularly getting less than seven hours of
sleep per night, which places them (or you) at increased
risk for early brain aging, muscle and joint breakdown—
and even becoming overweight. (I'll bet you never thought
your weight problem could be related to your lack of sleep!)

- The next two essential health components are the related
  issues of *diet* and *nutrition*. Two-thirds of our nation's
  adult population is overweight or obese, and even though
  we don't look like it from the outside, many are actually
  malnourished—living primarily on "empty calories."
  Most every common disease is somehow related to your
  food intake and weight distribution—so it is critically
  important that you know the best way to care for yourself
  in these areas.

- The fourth and fifth areas address your body's bone and
  muscle health, as these body parts are primarily responsible for moving you around in this life. Acquiring proper
  posture and possessing adequate *strength and flexibility* are crucial if you are to recover from, or avoid, many
  orthopedic-type physical disabilities, such as herniated
  discs, arthritis, and tendonitis.

- Finally, you need to know how to maximize your *brain
  health* so you can guard against premature brain aging.
  I'm sure you want your mind to remain sharp and clear for
  as long as you live, just like I do. Research shows that brain
  deterioration actually begins after your thirtieth birthday!

  According to studies conducted at Rush Medical Center in Chicago, roughly *50 percent* of people who reach 85
  will develop dementia. Yet here is the reason to have hope:
  There are many lifestyle changes you and I can make that
  are proven to support the health of our brains and positively
  impact our memory and ability to think analytically long
  into our golden years. Remember, Moses was 120 years old

and he was still governing the nation of Israel. (And if you think that happened only in biblical times, my husband's grandmother is still as sharp as a tack—and she's 100.)

Making a Start

If we all could compare notes, we would find that each one of us struggles with different areas of our health—and to different degrees. Someone might need a simple tune-up, while another might require a major health overhaul. Many of you would admit that you could use some help in *all six* of these health components.

If you are in this latter group, determine not to become overwhelmed by trying to make adjustments in every area of your life all at the same time. To be successful over the long haul, you must view wellness as a *journey*, not a destination. And no one's expecting you to turn into an Olympic athlete. Instead, this book is filled with straightforward, easy-to-apply health "nuggets," which when put into practice, promise to make big changes in your health today, tomorrow, and throughout your lifetime.

In part 2 you'll find these six wellness areas laid out smorgasbord style. This way you can pick and choose, digging in to the specific areas you wish to improve. As you make gains in one area, turn your attention to working on another component of your self–health care plan. And if an area where you've made progress begins to slide (as regular exercise does with me), simply begin again. Past failures do not predict future ones. Truthfully, failure can actually teach you what method doesn't work for you. Let's agree right here to not give up on our pursuit of better health!

● ● ●

Are you ready to invest in your future, my friend? Can you be described by the well-known phrase: "sick and tired of being sick and tired"? Or do you want to ensure that—as far as it depends on you—you'll do everything you can to not become worn out as the years progress? If you are concerned that declining health, a depleted energy level, or a foggy brain might stand between you and what you believe God wants you to do, then take this invitation from me to rebuild and protect your health. I'll be with you on the journey.

But before we get down to the actual business of rebuilding, let's first get our firm foundation poured directly from Scripture. This way we can make sure our hearts, minds, and souls are rightly aligned with God's will for our wellness.

LET'S REVIEW

1. Investing in your wellness will yield great dividends not only in this life, but for all eternity.

2. We are called Christ's ambassadors here on earth.

3. Yet the church has become indistinguishable from the world when it comes to obesity, disability, and disease-by-choice.

4. The systematic breakdown of a believer's body effectively, and progressively, reduces his or her usefulness in serving as Christ on this earth.

5. There is much that you can do to resist, reverse, and reconstruct the aging process.

6. Past failures in improving your health do not predict future ones.

7. Are you ready to start taking better care of the wonderful gift God has given you—your body? If so…let's go!

②

Why Be Well?

Your God-Planned Itinerary

We are God's workmanship, created in Christ Jesus to
do good works, which God prepared in advance for us to do.

EPHESIANS 2:10

You and I live in the information generation, where we are continually bombarded with health messages that encourage us to do such things as "Eat more fruits and vegetables"; "Sleep seven to eight hours a night"; "Strengthen your abdominal core muscles." In addition, headlines and taglines keep us informed of the latest statistics regarding declining health within our nation: "Two of three American adults are overweight, one in three people over the age of 20 have prediabetes or full-blown diabetes; heart disease is now the number-one killer in the US." This overload of advice and warnings has left many of us jaded. There is so much we *should* do that we become overwhelmed and do nothing.

The Right Kind of Willpower

Those of you who have sought to heed those health warnings and change your ways have likely found that your success in doing the healthier thing was relatively short-lived and ultimately ended in frustration and defeat. I find there are typically two reasons for this less-than-desired result.

The first is that your motivation to make a change was likely fueled by personal ambition. You see, if your health goals are *temporal* (to fit into your jeans, lower your cholesterol, or feel better), then your results will likely be *temporary*. Even desiring to live long enough to watch your grandchildren grow up (a noble aspiration) does not provide adequate inspiration to consistently maintain a lifestyle that favors longevity. For years I have watched people make bad choices during their thirties and forties that drive their health into the ground during the second half of their life—all because they fail to see their life's purpose from a heavenly perspective.

The second reason you may have experienced repeated failure when trying to improve or maintain better health is because you've relied solely upon your own willpower. I'm sure you'd agree that your power to motivate yourself is finite. We humans are fickle. Our passion for positive change rises and falls—often with the seasons. The warmer the weather, the less we are covered up, and the more motivated we are to get in shape. No wonder we experience on-again, off-again results.

For instance, I have four friends who have gained and lost over 70 pounds. Two have kept the weight off, and the other two regained their weight in a matter of a year. What is the difference? According to Scripture, only God can provide us with the continual willpower we need to accomplish what He has intended for us—*His will*, and the *Holy Spirit's power*. My two friends who have continued to maintain a healthy weight view their diet and exercise programs as part of a spiritual battle. My other two friends just wanted to look and feel better—and they did, but for only a short while.

If we are to stay on the path toward improved health and wellness, we need to change our focus, our goal, and our motivation. We must fix our eyes heavenward and begin to concentrate on what God wants and desires for us. Many of you will be surprised at how much the Scripture has to say when it comes to your physical health and wellness. Usually the best place to start an investigation is at the beginning—but for our purposes today, we'll need to start *before* the beginning…

Before You Were Born

If you received the same sort of public school education I did, you were led to believe that you came into being by way of millions of years of happenstance mutations. Thankfully, at the same time I was receiving *that* version, I was getting a completely different explanation (from my parents and my Sunday school teachers) as to how and why I came to be—*God's will.* The Bible is exceedingly clear on this: You and I were created by God, in His image, for His good pleasure…and we were fully known by Him *before we were even born.* Before a single day of your life came to pass, you were intimately known and fully planned for and by God. Here's the testimony of Scripture:

- *King David:* "When I was woven together in the depths of the earth, your eyes saw my unformed body. All the days ordained for me were written in your book before one of them came to be" (Psalm 139:15-16).

- *The prophet Isaiah:* "Before I was born the Lord called me…" (Isaiah 49:1), and "…he…formed me in the womb to be his servant" (Isaiah 49:5).

- *God (speaking to Jeremiah):* "Before I formed you in the womb I knew you, before you were born I set you apart; I appointed you as a prophet to the nations" (Jeremiah 1:5).

- *The apostle Paul:* "We are God's workmanship, created in Christ Jesus to do good works, which God prepared in advance for us to do" (Ephesians 2:10).

That last verse has really made me pause to think. God has prepared good works for us to do…in advance. In advance of what? Why, in advance of our own creation! Really think about that. Before your debut on Planet Earth, your Creator already had your unique blueprints in hand and had specific tasks planned for you to complete. And guess what He gave you to use while you go about fulfilling your "heavenly to-do list"? You guessed it—your well-tuned body. (Okay, so it used to be well-tuned…)

MAKING TIME FOR GOD'S AGENDA

Judging by the length of your to-do list these days, you must already be accomplishing many of those God-ordained good works—yes? Well, maybe not as much as you think. A few years back, when I began to realize that I couldn't accomplish all that was on my calendar (and still maintain a peaceful spirit), God stepped in with some redirection for me that I'd like to share with you.

Is it possible that your schedule is loaded up with tasks that might not be the good works God has intended for you? Oh sure, they might all be good tasks—but are they *God*-tasks? Sometimes we Christians feel compelled to fulfill the needs at our church or within our communities without asking God's opinion first. And because we load up our schedules by doing good we can often fail to accomplish the unique purposes for which God has designed (and predestined) us. I have no doubt that there is enough time in every day to do what God wants us to do. (Remember, it was He who came with up a 24-hour day minus the 7 to 8 hours we need to spend looking at the back of our eyelids.) It is our job as Christ-followers to make sure we don't miss our pre-planned appointments.

The way I now go about determining what to say yes to and what to decline, is that whenever a request is made for my time, I bring it before the Lord in prayer and ask for His direction. I also run it by the spiritual head of my home—my husband. And as a rule of thumb, I never add something onto my schedule without off-loading another thing. In addition, I periodically pray through my scheduled commitments to make sure my days are spent answering God's call and not man's.

Your Body, *His* Temple

On the day you were born, God gave you the keys to a new motor home—your earthly body. As planned by God, your "motor home" is your only form of transportation this side of heaven. The day you became a follower of Jesus Christ, your vehicle received an upgrade (a conversion package, if you will). Penned across the back of your vehicle in fancy lettering is your new road name: *The Temple of the Holy Spirit*. I'm not making this up—well, at least not the part about the conversion package. Look at what Paul writes in 1 Corinthians 6:19:

> Do you not know that your body is a temple of the Holy
> Spirit, who is in you, whom you have received from God?

When Paul stated this fact, it was a new revelation for the early church. You see during Old Testament times, God's Spirit resided primarily within the temple building itself—or more specifically, within an inner room of the temple called the holy of holies. Once a year, on the Day of Atonement (Yom Kippur), the high priest of Israel was allowed to enter this most holy of rooms. And although he was surrounded by the Holy Spirit's presence within the holy of holies, he was never filled internally with it.

On a few occasions we find that the Holy Spirit would temporarily "rest upon" or even "fill" an individual such as Moses or David. However, the allotment of the Holy Spirit changed radically when, at the exact time of Christ's death, the curtain (veil) that separated the holy of holies (and thus the Holy Spirit) from the worshippers of God was torn in two, from top to bottom. This miraculous act symbolized, among other things, that the Holy Spirit's presence would no longer be exclusive—reserved for a privileged few. Through Christ's perfectly redemptive sacrifice, God was now able to commune with His people in an up close and personal way.

Fifty days later, on the day of Pentecost, this became clearly evident as every individual believer that day was filled with the Holy Spirit. From that time until today, everyone who calls on the name of the Lord Jesus Christ is not only saved from the penalty of his sins, but is also filled with the Holy Spirit. And for the first time in Scripture, the body of one of God's people is called a *temple of the Holy Spirit*.

Viewing your physical body as a temple of the Holy Spirit is a vital perspective for you to have before embarking on a new journey toward better health. It will serve to anchor your determination to get well and stay well on something far more substantial than your own desires and good intentions. Throughout history the people of Israel meticulously built, rebuilt, and cared for the temple building where their God was known to dwell. They did this out of a sense of love, honor, and duty for the Lord. Striving to keep our "temples" in good shape also reflects our love and devotion to the Lord. Allow this to sink in: as a Christian the Spirit of God *lives* within your body. I believe that if you are consistently mindful of the awesome privilege you've been given, you will feel compelled to do some "home repairs" and sprucing up.

Your body, *His* temple. Your responsibility, *His* power. How wonderful it is to be partnered with the Lord!

You Are Not Your Own

Each year—for *my* birthday—I enjoy hosting my friends for a Victorian tea party. (I know that sounds backward, but it's a great blessing to *be* a blessing.) One year I asked my mother-in-law if I could borrow her antique knobbed milk-glass rose bowl for the center of the table. From all the words I used to properly describe it, you can sense that it was old and rare (and expensive)—but I was doing a white table theme and was willing to take the risk of having it in my possession (with my two kids bounding around my home) for the week.

Well, you'd better believe I took extra good care of that rose bowl! I lifted it just so, set it down gently, and made sure I wrapped it up safely when I was finished using it. I did all that care taking because the rose bowl was not mine—it was merely on loan to me. More importantly, I knew how much my mother-in-law loved that glass piece. It would sadden her greatly if I were to damage or destroy it—not to mention how difficult and costly it would be to replace.

My friend, you and I are like that cherished rose bowl in God's eyes. Consider Paul's statement in the second sentence of 1 Corinthians 6:19:

> You are not your own; you were bought at a price.

Just like that valuable bowl didn't belong to me, your precious body is not your own to do with as you please. Furthermore, you were bought at an exorbitantly high price—Christ's blood shed on the cross. If our aim is to be good stewards of the bodies on loan to us, then we have no other choice than to manage our temples with great care. Similar to honoring God with your other gifts (skills, time, and wealth) you must decide to honor Him with the way you care for and protect His purchased treasure—your physical body.

Choosing to Honor God

If I asked you if you thought you should honor God, I bet you'd answer without hesitation, "Of course I should!" If I then followed up by asking you, "Do you honor God *with your body?*" your response would likely be more hesitant. "Well...I try to...but I guess I don't always...I mean, there's always room for improvement, right?" That is a respectable answer because, truthfully, it is the response every person should give. None of us have arrived when it comes to this multifaceted health-care task. Honoring God with your body is a daily, and sometimes hourly, choice each of us has to make. In the concluding sentence of 1 Corinthians 6:19 Paul lets us know that honoring the Lord with our physical being is a command:

Therefore honor God with your body.

Just what exactly does it mean to honor God with your body? If I asked my son's Sunday school class they would likely offer answers such as "You can honor God with your body by not using your hands to steal or to hit someone." Being teenage boys (with the opposite sex on their minds with increasing regularity) they might also answer that you should not be sexually active outside marriage and that you should make sure that your eyes don't look at unholy images—movies, magazines, Internet sites. Likely most Christians, young and old, would list off many of the same answers to that very question. Yet there is another critical aspect of honoring God with your body, which should rank near the top of your list. It is the physical care of your body, His temple.

As we discussed back in the introduction, you were created to use your hands and your feet (your physical being) on this earth for a divine purpose—to serve the bride of Christ (the church) and those who are not yet saved (the world). Only by taking the steps needed to get healthier and remain well can you succeed in living out your intended role in God's plan for the people around you. There is only one you, and your unique, predetermined tasks can only be performed *by you*. In the same way that my children choose to honor me with their bodies when they do what I've asked them to do—take out the trash, fold the laundry, wash the car—you and I can honor God by being ready, willing, and *able* to do what He asks of us. When we seek to age well, live long, and serve strong we demonstrate great honor for our King!

Obeying Jesus' #1 Commandment

When a Pharisee asked Jesus to define what the most important commandment in all of Scripture was, He replied,

> Love the Lord your God with all
> your heart, soul, mind, and *strength*.
> Mark 12:30

In this statement Jesus gave a "Cliff Notes version" of the first four commandments found in the book of Exodus in the Old Testament, which serve to govern our relationship with God. If we strive to obey all of Jesus' primary command (and God's top four commandments), then it is crucial that we understand what it is that Christ requires of us. So let's dissect this verse.

The first component, loving God with *all your heart*, covers the area of your emotions—joy, passion, awe, and so on. By nature most Christians do not struggle with loving the Savior with their heartfelt emotions.

Secondly, *all your soul* refers to your eternal being, which resonates with God's eternal nature—at the time of your salvation your spirit connected with God, and you were sealed with His Holy Spirit. This act of becoming one with the Godhead enables you to love the Lord with your soul, or your spiritual-eternal being.

The third way we are instructed to love God is with *all our minds*, the source of our thought life. We can demonstrate our love for God in this third way by focusing our minds on righteous, holy, truth-filled thoughts, and by meditating on His holy Word. Not surprisingly this is an area where Satan loves to attack. As a result, trying to love God in this third way can get awfully polluted with "stinking thinking." I spend an entire chapter in my book *Overcoming Overeating* helping readers learn how to train their minds away from thinking thoughts that are destructive and replace them with thoughts that are constructive.

So what does Jesus have in mind when He asks us to love God with *all of our strength*? Here is where we talk about physical effort. The church has been awfully quiet when it comes to the act of loving God with our personal physical health and wellness. Could it be that the commandment is fulfilled by giving God whatever physical effort we can muster—even if it is meager because we're not feeling so well these days? Maybe we shouldn't put emphasis on the word "all," but rather be satisfied with "some" or "whatever remains."

I have a hard time accepting those explanations. The real reason I believe that loving God with *all* of our physical strength is often brushed aside is because it requires effort and consistent discipline. But the undeniable fact is that Jesus calls us to love God fully in all four areas. We do not get to pick and choose.

Physical Worship

Before we move on to the nuts and bolts of how to go about restoring and maintaining better health, think about this: Taking care of your physical body is an act of *worship*. Look at Paul's words in Romans 12:1:

> I urge you, brothers, in view of God's mercy, to
> offer your bodies as living sacrifices, holy and pleasing
> to God—this is your spiritual act of worship.

When you concentrate some of your efforts on restoring and maintaining your health, you are presenting your body to God as a living sacrifice, and in doing so, you worship God. Any other motivation you attempt to use to bring about change will fall far short of this one.

Remember, we need to hold on to an incentive that is greater than the temporal and that will remain consistent over time.

In the original text of the New Testament, the word translated repeatedly as "worship" in our English Bibles is actually two unique Greek words that have different meanings. The first word that is translated "worship" is *proskuneo* (pronounced pros-koo-NEH-o), which literally means to "bow the knee" or "bow down before." This is the reverent posture we display before our King. We worship God in the *proskuneo* way when we bow our heads, bend our knees, or outright prostrate ourselves before the Lord, honoring His supremacy.

The second Greek word translated in the Bible as "worship" is *latreuo* (pronounced lat-ROO-o) or *latreia* (lat-RAY-ah). It is this word we find used in Romans 12:1 when Paul speaks of our "spiritual act of worship." *Latreia*, which is best defined "to labor for or serve," reflects an *active* form of worship. Paul is urging us to worship God by laboring as His ambassadors in service to the church and in ministry to the world. When we offer our bodies up to God in this way, as a living sacrifice, we should also be saying: *Lord, I will make the sacrifices necessary to maintain a body that is ready, willing, and able to serve you.*

When we are saddled with a neglected, abused body rather than a strong, ready-for-service Holy Spirit temple, our spiritual act of worship for the Lord is most certainly diminished. Thankfully, we can make steps to turn that situation around by deciding to worship God with the food we eat, the length of time we sleep, and by the way in which we keep our minds and our muscles ready for action. Caring for the condition of your body for the purpose of serving Christ is true worship!

● ● ●

We've laid a lot of groundwork here in this chapter. This issue of personal health has taken on much greater dimensions, hasn't it? You can begin to see your life and your health from a divine vantage point. As you journey toward a healthier and more productive future, which includes better sleeping, eating, posture, and exercising habits, I am convinced that this biblical motivation will prove itself to be as powerful in your life as it has in my own.

With this spiritual perspective in place, let's move ahead to the next chapter. From studying the Old Testament book of Nehemiah, I have uncovered some principles that can be incredibly transforming when applied to the restoration of your temple!

LET'S REVIEW

1. You will be hard-pressed to make lasting health changes without an accurate spiritual perspective of your life.

2. Forget about mustering up your own willpower; rather seek God's *will* and the Holy Spirit's *power*.

3. God planned works for you to do before you were even born—be ready to participate!

4. If you are a believer, your "earthly tent" houses the Holy Spirit.

5. Your body is owned by God. He desires to use *your* hands and feet to accomplish *His* kingdom work. Your life was planned for such a time as this.

6. Honoring God with your body, through the stewardship of your health, demonstrates your love for the Lord and is a bona fide spiritual act of worship.

A Biblical Blueprint for Restoration

The 7-Step Plan for Renewing Your Health

O Lᴏʀᴅ my God, I cried to you for help,
and you restored my health.

PSALM 30:2 NLT

When I began thinking about the topic of restoring physical health, I started by reading the Old Testament account of Nehemiah's rebuilding of the walls around the city of Jerusalem because it is the best known biblical account of "restructuring." What God revealed to me that day left my heart racing and my mouth hanging open—there before my own eyes, within the first few chapters of the book of Nehemiah, was a completely applicable blueprint that outlined a step-by-step plan for restoration. Without variation of even a single point, it gave perfect direction for those of us who want to re-establish our physical well-being!

Throughout the remainder of this chapter I will show you how to apply each of these vital steps—in the same order that Nehemiah used them—which I trust will result in a God-empowered, Spirit-led rejuvenation of your health and wellness. For those of you who are unfamiliar with the book of Nehemiah or would like a quick refresher, you can get quickly up to speed by reading chapters 1–4 and 6. If you don't have a Bible within reach, I'll begin with a short story version.

Meet Nehemiah

The year was 445 BC, roughly 70 years after the end of the Babylonian captivity of the nation of Israel (which itself lasted 70 years). During those 70 years the previously exiled people of Israel had slowly begun to return to their hometown of Jerusalem. As this account begins, Nehemiah, one of the Jewish exiles, was serving as the cupbearer for King Artaxerxes, the king of Persia.

One day while Nehemiah was in the king's palace, his brother, along with some other trusted Israelite friends, came to see him. These men had just returned from Judah—the province where the holy city of Jerusalem was located. Their beloved city was in dire condition. The high, protective walls that used to surround the city had lain demolished for more than a century, and the city's many gates had been burned with fire. Oh, how could the once thriving city of Jerusalem—which housed the very Spirit of the Almighty in its holy temple—have been brought so low? Overwhelmed by this troubling report, Scripture tells us that Nehemiah sat down and wept bitterly.

The many years that Nehemiah spent in exile had not diminished his passion for Jerusalem—the very city in which God had chosen to reside—or for his fellow countrymen. He grieved desperately, not only because he was embarrassed that his nation's actions had led to the destruction of the Lord's temple, but also because he knew that the Israelites who were returning to that city were in a position of vulnerability and disgrace. Nehemiah knew that without Jerusalem's walls and gates intact, the city and its people lived in grave danger. Worse still, the once great nation of Israel, along with their God, was being mocked by their neighbors. God's chosen people were forced to live with their heads hung in shame.

Nehemiah was most definitely a man of action. But he was first and foremost a man of prayer. Immediately after receiving the dreadful news of his beloved city's ruin, Nehemiah spent days repenting and petitioning the Lord. It was during that vulnerable time that God placed a desire deep within his heart to rebuild the walls of Jerusalem for the purposes of restoring her protection and erasing her shame.

God's Provision

Nehemiah knew it would be a God-sized task to rebuild God's favorite city. So he asked one last thing of the Lord. He asked Him for success. And God showed Himself strong in the weeks and months that followed. One day King Artaxerxes asked his cupbearer about the sadness that was written across his face. When Nehemiah came forward with the whole story, including his plan to rebuild the city's walls and gates, the king did not hesitate to grant him everything he asked for—and then some. A leave of absence from his job as cupbearer, sufficient timber to build with, a small army of soldiers to keep him safe on his journey, "letters of recommendation"—you name it, God provided it through the king!

If your health is presently in disrepair, right from the outset of your journey both you and Nehemiah likely share many of the same emotions. Has God placed a similar desire within your heart today—to rebuild your health and restore His temple? If you're tired of feeling ashamed about your body and the state it is in, and you sense that you may be at high risk for sickness, injury, or disease, then you are standing in a very promising place—on the threshold of renewed health! As we move through the rest of this chapter I will show you exactly how each step that Nehemiah used from concept to completion can be used to not only restore, but also to maintain good health on into your golden years.

Nehemiah's 7-Step Plan

Nehemiah's approach to rebuilding the walls around Jerusalem provides a perfect blueprint for achieving your own goal of improved personal health. You'll find there is spiritual wisdom as well as practical significance in the sequence of steps. Now let's gather our wisdom, direction, and motivation straight from Scripture, beginning this journey of rebuilding your health right where Nehemiah did…on his knees.

STEP ONE: Cry Out to the Lord

When Nehemiah received that awful report that day in the palace, the Bible describes his response in just one powerful verse:

> When I heard these things, I sat down and
> wept. For some days I mourned and fasted
> and prayed before the God of heaven.
>
> NEHEMIAH 1:4

Many years ago I received the heart-shattering news that my then 11-year-old daughter was suffering from an auto-immune illness called Graves' disease. We were given 50-50 odds for her cure. Her treatment would require a regimen of multiple pills taken four times a day, likely for two years. (At one point she was up to 11 pills a day.) My world became filled with what ifs and what-thens. Our weeks were scheduled with blood draws and medical appointments with her endocrinologist and cardiologist. My sweet, once-healthy daughter had a serious disease! Brokenhearted, I mourned and fasted and prayed, continually bringing my request for her recovery before the Lord. God acted mightily...and in His time, my daughter was healed!

Where are you today? Are you grieving the loss of your own health? Have you gotten to the point where you are ready to cry out to the Lord? If so, then please know that God is grieving right alongside you. He is your Creator and your loving Father. It saddens Him deeply to watch your health slip away, just as it troubled me to watch my daughter's once perfect body be taken over by disease.

If you want to make lasting changes to improve your health, begin exactly where Nehemiah did—with a desperate cry. Go ahead, cry out to the Lord. Allow yourself to grieve your present condition and your past choices. This needs to be your first step on the road to recovery and restoration. A desperate cry to the Lord works to open your spiritual ears. C.S. Lewis said, "God whispers to us in our pleasures, speaks to us in our conscience, but shouts in our pain: it is His megaphone to rouse a deaf world." May we be so roused!

STEP TWO: Seek His Forgiveness

The second step in the Bible's blueprint for restoring your health is this: You must be willing to confess your sin and take ownership of your disobedience. The Bible makes it clear that allowing your health to deteriorate because of neglect or abuse *is* sin. Proverbs 23:2 and verses 20-21 speak of the sin of excessive food and drink (gluttony and drunkenness). But can't neglect of exercise be seen as a sin too? (I am paying close attention to this one myself.) When it comes to this, most of us would admit that we are often just plain lazy. And the Bible has much to say about laziness. In fact the book of Proverbs contains 14 comments about lazy people (sluggards), none of which are glowing! So while it is not called a sin, the attitude of laziness is most certainly given the thumbs-down.

Your spiritual rebirth began with your sincere confession and repentance. So, too, seeking to have your health reborn must begin in the same way. Scripture tells us that Nehemiah demonstrated his confession and repentance by mourning, fasting, and praying. Through his tears (of sincerity), he openly confessed his sin (his responsibility) before the Lord, and sought the Lord for a way to make things right again (atonement) for the nation of Israel. If we are to successfully regain and maintain our vitality, we must approach the throne of our Maker and take full responsibility for the things we have done (or not done) that have left our bodies prematurely vulnerable to sickness or disability. Then we must determine not to continue walking the same path. This restorative repentance will allow us to honestly dedicate ourselves to making things right—as far as it depends on us.

BETTER HEALTH, NOT PERFECT HEALTH

Throughout this whole process, keep in mind that you are on your way to better health, not perfect health. We must pursue it in the same way we seek to live holy lives: a little more each day, one good choice at a time, experiencing failures along the way, demonstrating repentance, and receiving forgiveness. And even with all the ups and downs we will inevitably experience, if we remain determined, our journey will be characterized by forward momentum, increasingly enjoying more of what God wants for us!

STEP THREE: Ask for His Empowerment

Restoring your health will mean fighting an uphill spiritual battle as well as a physical battle. Remember, Satan is quite content to have you sitting on the sidelines of service, functioning below the level of your calling. So exactly how will you be able to move forward in this battle if you already feel defeated? You need to go before God and ask Him to empower you—just as Nehemiah did.

The third step in remodeling your health is found in Nehemiah's prayer requests in chapter 1, verse 11:

> O Lord, let your ear be attentive to the prayer of this your
> servant and to the prayer of your servants who delight in
> revering your name. Give your servant success today…

Nehemiah knew exactly what he needed to move forward in what God was calling him to do. He realized he would never be successful unless God empowered him. The power to reform your ways, to make healthy choices, and to pursue healing must come from God Himself. God will always grant us the power to do that which is according to His will—and by now I hope you are convinced that your improved health is most certainly God's will for you. And the wonderful thing is that all you have to do is ask for success. The power of the Holy Spirit is yours each new day.

I'll bet you are in the same boat as I am—lacking the ability to do great and lasting things on your own. Renowned evangelist R.A. Torrey had a keen insight into the power of prayer:

> The reason why many fail in battle is because they wait
> until the hour of battle. The reasons why others succeed
> is because they have gained their victory on their knees
> long before the battle came…Anticipate your battles, fight
> them on your knees *before temptation comes*, and you will
> always have victory.

Torrey gives us invaluable advice here—to anticipate the challenges and pray *before* they begin. When it comes to spiritual warfare, *prayer equals power, and power equals success.* We would be ill-equipped to step into this battle without prayer. We all know people (including ourselves) who have begun a diet, started a new exercise program, or made a healthy New Year's resolution. Fast-forward a year. How many have kept it up? The reason we are unsuccessful in the long term is because we do not apply this third step—we try to accomplish change on our own strength. Let's take to heart the words of Torrey and depend on God's might and not our own.

STEP FOUR: Take an Honest Assessment of Your Health

With steps one through three behind him, Nehemiah was on to step four, making a detailed assessment of the situation at hand:

> I set out during the night with a few men. I had not told anyone what my God had put in my heart to do for Jerusalem. There were no mounts with me except the one I was riding on.
>
> By night I went out through the Valley Gate toward the Jackal Well and the Dung Gate, examining the walls of Jerusalem, which had been broken down, and its gates, which had been destroyed by fire. Then I moved on toward the Fountain Gate and the King's Pool, but there was not enough room for my mount to get through; so I went up the valley by night, examining the wall. Finally, I turned back and reentered through the Valley Gate. The officials did not know where I had gone or what I was doing, because as yet I had said nothing to the Jews or the priests or nobles or officials or any others who would be doing the work.
>
> NEHEMIAH 2:11-16

This next step of careful inspection took place *privately* between Nehemiah and his God. While you are reading through this book, assessing the damage in your "walls and gates," I suggest that you privately and prayerfully consider your findings, getting ready for later action.

Have you ever been involved in a building or remodeling project? I remember when my husband and I set out to add just 300 square feet to our first home. The preconstruction, planning stage seemed to take as long as the building project itself. We had to first adequately assess the present condition of our home along with our available funds. Only then could we intelligently reconcile the realities of finances (our present) with our desires for the future.

Similarly, when setting out to restore your health, you need to begin by making a thorough appraisal of your present health condition, comparing it to what you'd like it to be in the future. With that assessment in place you will be able to construct a specific, prioritized plan of action which takes into account where you are now. (Chapters 4–9 contain the tools you'll need to do that.) When you have undergone a thorough "health inspection," then you can move from the stage of private planning into the public realm.

STEP FIVE: Verbalize Your Commitment to Change

With a full understanding of all that needed to be done, and with the assurance that he had the supplies that would be required, Nehemiah finally made his intentions public.

> Then I said to them, "You see the trouble we are in:
> Jerusalem lies in ruins, and its gates have been burned
> with fire. Come, let us rebuild the wall of Jerusa-
> lem, and we will no longer be in disgrace." I also told
> them about the gracious hand of my God upon me
> and what the king had said to me. They replied, "Let
> us start rebuilding." So they began this good work.
>
> Nehemiah 2:17-18

Nehemiah knew that if the city's walls and gates were to be restored, he'd need to tell the people of Jerusalem what God was leading him to do. He also had to enlist their help. The same is true for you. When you reach the point where you are ready to begin your own rebuilding project, don't just try to renew your health quietly (and hope no one notices when you backslide). Make a declaration! Announce the plan

God has laid on your heart—to restore your health for the sake of His kingdom. Tell your spouse, your kids, your family, your close friends—even your co-workers. This will help to solidify your decision to move forward in this area of your life.

A few years ago, during my quiet time, God specifically spoke to me telling me it was "time to write." To which I nervously replied; "Write what?" He eventually revealed to me that He wanted me to write a book which would help to physically restore His people and enable them to perform the kingdom works He had planned for them. I was less than prepared to write a book...where does one even start? Not to mention that my father, whose education included a master's degree in English literature, had convinced me way back when I was a teenager that I had no talent when it came to writing. I didn't want to risk the embarrassment of failure, and I wasn't quite sure I wanted all that work!

But I *knew* God had called me to write, and I always told the Lord that whenever I heard His voice, I would obey. Even so, I was well aware of my human nature. I could easily talk myself out of this book-writing thing without anyone ever knowing. So I did what I knew from experience needed to be done in order to cement God's call on my life: I told someone. And not just anyone—I told someone who I knew would remind me of my declaration and keep me accountable.

STEP SIX: Develop a Detailed Plan of Action

Nehemiah's preconstruction phase, in which he took careful inventory of each section of broken wall and burnt gate that would need to be repaired, led to the formation of a specific action plan. Throughout chapter 3 of his book, Nehemiah records in great detail exactly who was assigned to rebuild each section of the wall or reconstruct which particular gate. Only with a well-thought-through approach could such a massive undertaking have been coordinated.

Step six in this process will require you to decide on your own personalized plan of action. I have done the research and have formulated what I believe are the most effective approaches you can follow to restore and maintain your health and wellness in those six critical health areas we touched on in chapter 1. Throughout the coming chapters I will offer many suggestions in the areas of rest, weight loss, nutrition, posture, strength and flexibility, and mental acuity—all of which will work together to restore your temple. Only you can decide which area needs the "first coat of paint." You have the freedom to choose whether you'll concentrate your efforts in one area at a time, or instead incorporate multiple changes in several areas at one time. Remember, this is *your* plan. Seek God (as Nehemiah did), and ask for His help prioritizing and determining the steps you should take.

STEP SEVEN: Use the Buddy System

In 1999 a popular British television game show began airing in the U.S.—*Who Wants to Be a Millionaire?* On the show, a contestant would answer a series of increasingly difficult questions, all in hopes of winning the grand prize of one million dollars. If stumped by a question along the way the contestant had three one-time "Lifelines" available to him: Fifty/Fifty (in which two of the four answer possibilities are eliminated from choice), Ask the Audience, or Phone-a-Friend. As you begin on this journey toward improved health, may I suggest that you Phone a Friend? A close friend can become an invaluable lifeline at times when you are tempted to give up on your revitalization process. Better yet, find a health-pursuing friend or mate and use the buddy system! Scripture promotes the use of a buddy system in Ecclesiastes 4:9-12, where Solomon observes,

> Two are better than one, because they have a good
> return for their work: If one falls down, his friend
> can help him up. But pity the man who falls and
> has no one to help him up!…Though one may
> be overpowered, two can defend themselves.

Nehemiah also knew the importance of a support system. He surrounded himself with like-minded people who shared the same vision: to see the walls of Jerusalem reconstructed. In fact, when enemy attack was feared, Nehemiah divided his workers into two groups; half continued to build while the other half stood ready to defend. My friend; Satan will try his best to attack and defeat you because he knows that a defeated Christian is of little use in the kingdom of God. So link spiritual arms with a buddy. Allow yourself to be held accountable and to be prayed for. Then press on toward the high calling of healthy living, all for His glory!

WALLS AND GATES

There is a marvelous analogy that can be drawn between the structural components that were rebuilt, the walls and the gates, and the main two choices you will face as you seek to restore your health.

Walls to Erect

The sole reason why walls were built around a city like Jerusalem was *to keep bad things out*. Likewise, you undoubtedly need to erect barriers or boundaries (walls) to prevent things from invading your life and negatively affecting your health. Without properly constructed "walls," our state of health is left vulnerable—open to attack, if you will.

In the third chapter of his book, Nehemiah lists each section of the wall and who was responsible for its repair. Think of each "section of the wall" in your own life to be a specific area of health you desire to restore. Wherever sections have fallen into disrepair over the years is where harmful "enemy attacks" come—and in many forms, such as eating diets high in saturated fats or simple carbohydrates, standing or sitting with slumped posture, living a life which lacks physical activity, and allowing the pace of your days to cheat you out of your much-needed sleep and leave you chronically exhausted.

Another thing to keep in mind about those walls is that watchmen were positioned along the top day and night so they could keep a lookout for any threat approaching. Likewise, you and I need to be "standing on top" of our newly erected walls, staying alert for those things that, if given access to our lives, would plunder our well-being.

Gates to Install

Gates, on the other hand, *allowed good things to enter* into the city.

Shepherds who grazed their flocks in the surrounding pastures had to enter the city to bring meat and milk, along with animals to be used for sacrificial purposes. Farmers needed to sell their produce in the marketplace. And those who tended orchards and vineyards had to enter through these gates with their harvest as well. Traveling merchants with goods to sell gained access to the city by its gates.

The gates allowed needful, life-giving supplies into the city. Part 2 of this book will suggest a whole host of things that we would be wise to "allow access" into our lives. Take this analogy one step further and think of each beneficial addition as a gate: advantageous things such as eating foods rich in fiber and anti-oxidants, maintaining proper postures, restoring strength and flexibility through exercises, performing mentally stimulating activities, and ensuring that we have adequate rest to meet the demands of our days.

Each chapter of part 2 covers one of the six foundations of good health: rest, weight loss, nutrition, posture, strength and flexibility, and brain function. In each case, I will point out to you specific "walls" that need to be fortified (or put into place), and which will provide significant protection against disease and disability. Also in each case, I will describe the best "gate" design for you to install to empower your pursuit of wellness. With strong walls and well-crafted gates in place, you can sleep easier (and hopefully longer), knowing you are protected and provided for in all the best ways!

A Time to Rejoice

In Nehemiah 6:15, we are given the final building report. The walls and gates of Jerusalem have been successfully restored. This marked a glorious time of new beginning for the people of Jerusalem. They celebrated this "new life" with songs of praise and by rededicating themselves to the Lord.

In part 2 of this book, I will show you how the seven-step plan for restoration can work in each of the six essential aspects of your well-being. When you've arrived at a place where you believe it is appropriate, may I suggest you rededicate your body to the Lord? By doing so you proclaim that you have chosen to be set apart for God's service, mind, body, and soul! Each of us at one time or another has desired a new beginning. Today is your chance for a fresh start.

> See, I am doing a new thing! Now it springs
> up; do you not perceive it? I am making a way
> in the desert and streams in the wasteland.
> ISAIAH 43:19

LET'S REVIEW

The Seven-Step Plan for Restoring Your Temple

STEP 1: Cry out to the Lord

STEP 2: Seek His forgiveness

STEP 3: Ask for His empowerment for success

STEP 4: Take an honest assessment of your health

STEP 5: Verbalize your commitment to change

STEP 6: Develop a detailed plan of action

STEP 7: Use the buddy system

PART 2

COMPONENTS OF ENDURING HEALTH

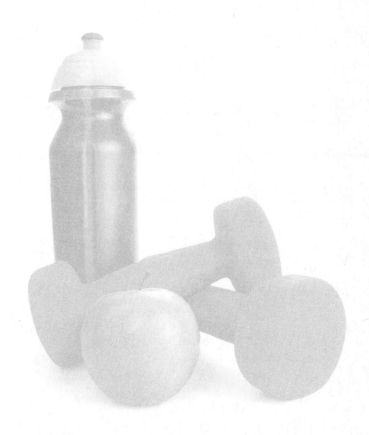

Rest for the Weary

The Truth About Sleep, Rest, and Recreation

Come to me, all you who are weary and burdened, and I will give you rest. Take my yoke upon you and learn from me, for I am gentle and humble in heart, and you will find rest for your souls.

MATTHEW 11:28-29

I have often heard the verse above quoted and honestly, I never really thought about the word "rest" (mentioned twice) as having anything to do with sleep. But it did make me think of something. Jesus was talking about rest being a great need of our hearts. It's also true that what a physically weary person needs most is rest—sleep! There are certainly many things in this life which come against us and make us feel tired to the bone: hard work, emotional strain, prolonged mental concentration, and so on. But I'm sure you'd agree that the thing that really does us in is a bad night's sleep...or, worse yet, multiple bad nights in a row!

When I was 13 or 14 years old, I remember going over to my best friend's house for a sleepover. Early in the evening we determined it would be so cool if we stayed up all night and watched the sun rise. Then we would have quite a tale to tell our friends when we returned to school on Monday morning! We were going strong until about 3 a.m. The next three hours were such a struggle. It felt like every fiber of my being longed for shut-eye. We did accomplish our goal that day (or early the following day)—but oh, the sleep deprived "hangover" we had to endure the next day! Even though I was a young, energetic (very energetic) teenager back then, it was all I could do just to drag myself through the next day. Have you ever had to pull an "all-nighter" in college or stay up all night with a sick child? Or maybe you can even relate to my teenage antics. You'd agree from experience that when we do not allow ourselves adequate sleep, we do not function as well as we could the next day.

God has created us with the need to sleep. You can only interfere with that requirement for so long before you begin to suffer. (This is the reason why sleep deprivation is often used as a form of torture.) If we're given the time and proper circumstances, we will sleep. But we must also pursue and protect our times of sleep, rest, and recreation if we are to maximize their benefits to our body, mind, and soul. Our bodies were built for function, but in order to maintain a highly functional life we must allow ourselves the opportunity to recharge.

What's So Important About Sleep?

I have met people throughout my life who love to brag about the fact they just don't *need* so much sleep. Their chests puff out as they proudly announce, "Five hours sleep—and I am good to go!" They feel sorry for all the rest of us less "evolved" people who have to "waste" so much of our time in Slumberville. Before I studied the subject of sleep and gained an understanding of all sleep had to offer, I must admit that I was somewhat jealous. I am a very productive person, and I would think to myself, *Wow, imagine what I could get done if I added another three hours to my day!* Well, I am no longer jealous—in fact I am saddened when I hear someone make the claim they can do fine on five hours of sleep. I am now fully aware of all the necessary components of good health they are getting only in short supply.

Sleep is not just the opposite of being awake, nor is it a state of simply being unconscious. It contains a vast treasure of good-for-you processes and necessary "manufacturing tasks" that assist your body in maintaining good physical and mental health throughout your lifetime. Dr. William Dement, cofounder of the Stanford University Sleep

Center, observes, "There is plenty of compelling evidence that *sleep* is the most important predictor of how long you will live."

So with all those health benefits to be had, it is awfully disturbing when studies show that *74 percent* of Americans don't get enough sleep at night. No wonder we are in such bad shape! I don't know what it is like where you live, but in my town they are erecting huge drugstores on every corner and on every available plot of land. And I don't think it is because we suddenly need more toilet paper. I believe it is the pharmaceutical industry that drives such expansion. We, as a nation, are excessively medicated! We are sold pills for everything that ails us— even lack of sleep. By the end of this chapter you will begin to see that getting a solid night's sleep can even help free you from needing some of your medications. Curious? I'll show you how.

The Architecture of Sleep

Even though we are all unique individuals, we do not vary greatly in our need for sleep. Current scientific studies still confirm that as adults we all need to sleep between 7 and 8 hours a night. No ifs, ands, or buts about it! Sleep requirements certainly do change from birth on into adulthood. When we are first born and our bodies are going through massive growth spurts (physically and neurologically), as babies we typically sleep 16 hours per day (not *mine,* though—which led to significant sleep deprivation for me!). Growing teenagers, who in my house seem to add an inch every two months to their height, require a solid 9 hours of sleep a night (yeah, mine seem to need 10...*now* they sleep!). But at 20 years of age on into our sunset years, our need for sleep decreases to 7 to 8 hours each night. In 2007 an important study out of London, England, showed that people who consistently slept *less than* or *more than* 7 to 8 hours per night showed a decreased life expectancy.

As a Christ-follower I am sure that you are keenly aware of His intricately amazing creative qualities. So it probably won't surprise you to find that your slumber has been designed in a divinely organized and purposeful way. Case in point: Not all sleep is the same. There are five stages of sleep you and I cycle through every 90 minutes or so as we are getting our shut-eye. We were designed to complete approximately five of these five-stage cycles per night, which adds up to seven-and-a-half hours. (I should have let you figure that out yourself. Computation is good food for your brain…more about brain health in chapter 9.)

Stage 1: Fragmented Sleep

When you lie down at night and close your eyes, if you're an average adult it could take upwards of 30 minutes to drift into this first stage. During stage 1 sleep you will tend to float in between being awake and being asleep; therefore it can be referred to as *fragmented sleep*. It is the shortest stage of the sleep cycle, lasting only five minutes or so. Often you'll succumb to stage 1 sleep at "non-bedtimes" such as while watching a boring movie, sitting through a long, drawn out meeting, or when listening to a sermon you've already heard before (but hopefully not when reading this book—unless it is very late at night, and then I beg you to put the book down and devote your attention to something more important—a good night's sleep!). As you know from experience, you can be easily roused when you have "fallen" into this stage—a little nudge or a whispered "wake up" will bring you right back to life!

Stage 2: Light Sleep

This second stage of sleep is the longest in duration, lasting from 40 to 50 minutes. It is best referred to as *light sleep* because, as with stage 1 sleep, you can be easily awakened when partaking in stage 2 slumber. It is during this stage that our body temperature drops, which scientists agree aids in the overall "sleepiness factor." (I bet God has an even more specific reason for this cool down; we just have yet to understand it.) Our core body temperature reaches its low point around 5 a.m., which for most people is about two hours before waking occurs. Older persons and those who suffer with chronic illnesses can spend their entire night in stage 2 sleep—further compounding their health issues (you'll discover why below)!

Stage 3: Deep Sleep

Now here is where we begin what is called "priority sleep" because as you'll soon see, our physical wellness depends upon it. The time spent in stage 3 is brief, lasting only 20 minutes. It is during this period that you have entered into *deep sleep* where arousal becomes more difficult. In stage 3 sleep your brain's activity changes dramatically from its stage 2 sleep pattern. It is also demonstrated to be *non-REM* sleep, which means that your eyeballs do not exhibit *rapid eye movement* (see below). In other words they slowly drift from side to side, scanning the back of your eyelids.

Stage 4: Very Deep Sleep

Similar to stage 3, this fourth stage lasts only 20 minutes and is characterized as non-REM sleep. Yet stage 4 sleep differs from stage 3 in the somewhat unique brain wave patterns it displays. Also known to be a priority form of sleep, stage 4 sleep must occur five times throughout the night in order for us to "milk it for all it's worth."

Stage 5: Dream State

This is the final stage of sleep that occurs before we start back again at stage 1. It lasts a mere five minutes—but make no mistake about it, this is a powerful five minutes! This stage is known as the *dream state* of sleep. During these five-minute bursts, our skeletal muscles become essentially paralyzed so we can't act out our dreams! (There is another interesting reason why this happens that we'll get to in a bit.) Stage 5 sleep is often referred to simply as REM sleep, as it is the only stage in which the body exhibits rapid eye movement. But of course—we have to watch all those dreams being played out before our eyes! In addition, stage 5 sleep brings a marked rise in blood pressure and pulse rate. I guess our dreams are just that exciting—even if we can't always remember them in the morning.

While You Were Sleeping...

Not only were we originally built by God, but He also designed us with a built-in way for our bodies to be repaired as we sleep. *Thank God for sleep!* many a weary person has said as they eased themselves into bed for the night. After you read about all the marvels of sleep's workings, you will be even more conscious of the thanksgiving we should offer Him for the part of our day of which we are least aware—sleep.

During *sleep stages 2 through 4* our bodies are busy mending our nervous system after an entire day of wear and tear. The nervous system is sort of like the body's electrical wiring. The "wires" (neurons) can get frayed, if you will, and in order to keep the electricity flowing, they need some repair work. After our neuroconnections have been fixed, they are sequentially tested to make sure everything is in working order.

Throughout *stages 3 and 4*, the deep and very deep non-REM stages of sleep, our bodies are busy building bone and muscle. This is a process that must continue throughout life even though the number of bones and muscles we have as adults don't change. God designed our bones to be in a continual state of breakdown and replacement—sort of like the roads and highways around New York City! Resistance training of any sort (yardwork, lifting weights) will send your brain messages to build bigger muscles—which is done primarily at night. As you can see, the very structure of our bodies depends on this most necessary phases of sleep.

Also of priority importance during these same two deep sleep phases is the replenishment of insulin (to control blood-sugar levels), growth hormone (to maintain muscle mass and skin integrity), and other neurotransmitters, such as serotonin, acetylcholine, dopamine, norepinephrine, and so on—each of which account for vital functions of your body and brain, as we'll discuss in more detail below.

Finally, during *stage 5 dream sleep,* or REM sleep—the phase during which our skeletal muscles are paralyzed—our skeletal muscle connections must be patched up because their fibers become damaged from daily use. (See the reason they had to be put to "sleep"? It is difficult to do "surgery" on a moving body.) And as with the neurologic components of our bodies, the repaired muscle fibers are tested to ensure a quick response when they are called on by the brain to move us about.

THINGS THAT WORK AGAINST
A GOOD NIGHT'S SLEEP ("WALLS")

Wondering why you can't fall asleep—or stay asleep at night? Here are a few quick fixes you can try. First of all, limit caffeine consumption to earlier in your day, say before 3 p.m. This includes caffeinated coffee, tea, soft drinks, and any form of chocolate, from hot chocolate to candy bars. Next you'll want to limit (or eliminate) evening alcoholic beverages. Alcohol has been shown to disrupt sleep patterns. Third, if you are taking antihistamines, you may want to consider a different approach to allergy control as medicines containing this component can really keep you up at night.

The Consequences of Sleep Deficiency

As I write this, my firstborn ("non-sleeping newborn") has just returned home from her day at high school. And even though 16 years have passed since her life's beginning I can still vividly remember what it was like to be thoroughly sleep-deprived! I should have known I was in trouble when, contrary to all the books I had read purporting that newborns sleep at least 16 hours a day (often in four-to-six hour stretches), my newborn took only 15-to-20 minute naps and then was happy and alert for the next five hours—ugh! It took Casey eight-and-a-half months to sleep through the night. That wouldn't have been so awful if she had awakened only once or twice a night during that period. But no, my sweet daughter was up, bright-eyed, four to five times a night. ("Night" in those days was from 11 p.m. to 5 a.m.—certainly shy of a full night.)

Recalling that time period in my life always makes me shudder. I got up each day in utter despair as my husband left for work—I was exhausted and the day (in which my young one would be up most the time) had just begun. My mood during that time was numb—neither happy nor depressed—just flat. I couldn't think clearly, speak fluently, or engage in lively conversation...I was just so tired! And the more tired I became, the less I could sleep.

Acute sleep deprivation is felt immediately upon rising to meet the new day. You feel groggy, unmotivated, and you drag yourself through the day wistfully hoping for another chance to sleep. Yet that is just the tip of the iceberg when it comes to the effects of chronic sleep deprivation on your body—which by definition is getting less than seven hours sleep per night over a prolonged period of time. There are a half dozen other things that are occurring, and once you are aware of them, that should be motivation enough to improve your sleep habits.

Weight Gain

I begin with this one because it is a consequence which most people have never heard of. Certainly if you are dragging through your day it would be reasonable to try to fuel yourself with quick energy food sources, which in turn could account for weight gain. Yet the problem is more intrinsic than that.

Deep in your brain, in the area now understood to be responsible for appetite control, you produce two opposing hormones. The first hormone is *leptin*, which has a *suppressing* effect on your appetite. The second hormone, *grehlin*, does exactly the opposite—it *stimulates* your hunger. When we are well-slept, our bodies produce normal amounts of both hormones. These hormones were created to work in tandem to let you know when you are hungry and when you have had enough. If, however, you allow yourself to fall into the pattern of getting a fewer number of these necessary sleep cycles each night, your brain will begin to *under*produce leptin and *over*produce grehlin. When this occurs not only will you lose your natural check on your appetite (leptin's job), but you will also find yourself hungrier throughout the day than you should be (due to excessive grehlin production).

Chronic sleep problems are also associated with increased production of *cortisol*, which recently has been widely advertised as one of the underlying factors in growing belly fat. So if your waistline is an issue for you, certainly modify your eating and exercise habits (as we'll discuss in upcoming chapters), but don't neglect getting adequate sleep. You need your hormones to work for you, not against you.

Acceleration of Aging

You know, it is harder being a woman in this society in many ways—one of which is this whole aging deal. We are bombarded with products to "reduce the effects of aging" from our skin. Magazines encourage us to get face lifts and tummy tucks, and to "lift" all the other areas that have fallen victim to gravity. No one lets you in on this little secret: *Get more sleep!* While you and I are spending time in stage 3 and 4 sleep, our brains are producing a very important chemical called *growth hormone.* And while we are no longer using this hormone to grow in stature, our bodies continue to use growth hormone to preserve the elasticity of our skin, strengthen our bones, and maintain good muscle mass. So if you used to laugh whenever your grandma said it was time she got her beauty sleep, you can stop laughing—Grandma was on to something.

Clouded Thinking

So many people go about their day in a sleep-deprived fog. We carry on, going about all our planned activities, and we never pause to wonder, *Hmmm, how capable am I, in this state, to do all that I am about to do?* Studies show sleep deprivation leads to an increase in traffic accidents and work related injuries.[1] We need to be aware that we are not "firing on all cylinders" and therefore, we must be extra careful if we know we haven't been sleeping all that well. One bad night's sleep is all it takes to alter our judgment and slow our reaction time. In fact, not enough sleep will also decrease your ability to do the following:[2]

- Make "executive" decisions
- Properly analyze information
- Form new memories (for example, *Where did I park my car/leave my keys?*)
- Access old memories

So if you are longing to clear those cobwebs from your mind and sharpen your mental "pencil," try a good night's sleep, 7 to 8 hours' worth.

Decline in Mental Health

In order to feel mentally well your brain needs access to a steady supply of a neurotransmitter called *serotonin.* Simply put, serotonin is a mood elevating chemical. Without adequate amounts you will begin to feel depressed, moody, and even anxious. Sadly, depression affects 6.7 percent of adults 18 years and older.[3] It is quite common for those suffering with depression to be diagnosed with a "chemical imbalance" (for example, not enough serotonin). In response to their paralyzing, mental health problem many have turned to prescribed pills just to make it through their day.

But what if those battling depression and other mental illnesses went back to basics and first tried to make more serotonin on their own before accepting help in the form of a pill? If a person can increase the time spent in the deep sleep stages 3 and 4 by getting a full night's sleep, they may be able to improve their own mood without becoming reliant on medication. It is certainly worth a try. Even if you still need to supplement your brain's own natural chemicals, possibly you'll find you can get by on a lower medicine dosage. (But never attempt to adjust your medication dosage without the supervision of your doctor.) And less medication is always better than more.

Weakened Immune System

Do you find yourself getting sick a lot? One cold ends and another begins, it seems—or maybe this time it's a stomach virus…While you may long for sleep when you are ill, maybe you have never thought that not getting enough sleep on all those nights when you're feeling well could be leaving you vulnerable for another illness, or even a dreadful disease. Numerous studies have confirmed that chronic "undersleepers" have significantly lowered immune responses. One study even clearly demonstrated that all it took to hamstring your immune system for the day was one five-hour night of sleep.[4] I had a friend and colleague who always prided himself on leading a very productive life on only five hours sleep a night. At 45 years old this otherwise healthy individual was diagnosed with lymphoma, and three months later he was in heaven. I have always wondered how big a role his lack of sleep played in his demise. I'll never know the answer, of course, but knowing what I now know about sleep and my immune system, as far as it depends on me, I will try to get my 7 to 8 hours of sleep each night.

Insulin Resistance

When you consistently find yourself cheating on sleep another undesirable effect is that your body's metabolism of sugar (a product of digested food) becomes inefficient. Every time you eat, your circulating blood sugar levels rise—which is expected. It is the job of your pancreas, through the production of the hormone insulin, to bring that rising sugar level back down into a normal range. The less time you spend in sleep stages 3 and 4, the less insulin your pancreas makes, and therefore the insulin that is available does a less-than-adequate job at controlling your blood sugar.[5] Add to this problem the fact that when your body is sleep-starved you also develop a decreased sensitivity to your own insulin...and you are up a sugary-sweet creek without a paddle.

If this subject is new for you, it's important to know that insulin resistance is the precursor for heart disease, stroke, diabetes, certain cancers, nerve damage, blindness, and so on. Too much is at stake not to know about this stealth robber of health for millions of people. My two previous books *Overcoming Overeating* and *Diabetes: Are You at Risk?* both provide a comprehensive overview.

Are you wondering if you can still keep up with all that needs to be done if you dedicate seven to eight hours to your pillow each night? Well, here's the catch—you'll lose all those hours you think you are gaining—in downtime caused by sickness, depression, injury, or disease. And there are fewer of God's planned works you are capable of doing with a broken-down body. So if you've decided that more sleep is what you need, let's proceed by going over a few good ways to get yourself ready for bed.

5 Steps to Get More Sleep Tonight

One of the best ways to ensure a good night's sleep is to plan for it. If your job allows (shift workers and moms of irregularly sleeping infants are excused), stick to a bedtime (lights out) and a morning wake time that are not widely varied. This means even on the weekends you should avoid staying up extra late and sleeping in. Your body has a natural sleep rhythm to it called the *circadian cycle*. This internal "human clock" repeats itself approximately every 24 hours. If you continually alter your sleep schedule, you wreak havoc with your body's own natural, chemically driven sleep cycle.

If falling asleep or staying asleep is a problem for you, here are a few aspects of better "bedroom hygiene":

1. *Keep your bedroom dark.* This means no falling or attempting to fall asleep with the television or other lights on. Interestingly, women are nine times more sensitive to light sources at night than men—so install light-proof window treatments in your room to avoid early morning sunrise wake-up calls.

2. *Keep your bedroom cool.* Your body's temperature drops during stage 2 sleep, which induces sleepiness. An overheated body tends not to stay asleep, as your core temperature is unable to decrease adequately. Yet a room that is too cold can also wake you up if you are shivering, feeling around for the covers your partner has kicked to the floor. The recommended room temperature is 65 to 72° F. But as with all things in life, what is good for the goose is not necessarily good for the gander. To solve this problem in my home, I bought a dual-setting electric blanket for the winter—so both my husband and I can achieve the sleeping temperature that best suits us.

3. *Keep your bedroom quiet.* Again, this means no television or loud music on. And put a hold on heavy, emotionally charged conversations right before going to bed—they can wait until morning.

4. *Invest in a good mattress and pillow.* Comfort is important when trying to sleep well. Sometimes it is not only the quality of your sleeping supplies, but the way you use them and position yourself at night that makes all the difference. If you are experiencing physical pain that either wakes you or keeps you from drifting off, get a copy of my book *Overcoming Back and Neck Pain.* Chapter 3 includes

a full discussion, complete with photographs, of healthy, pain-reducing or eliminating sleep postures.

5. *Reserve your bedroom for only two things: sleep and sex.* If you use your bedroom as an office or for television viewing, or if you bring your laptop in to search the web, then you will equate your bed/bedroom with mentally stimulating activities. This works against the soothing, sleep-inducing atmosphere it should be. The only exception to this rule is a little bit of pre-bedtime reading—but don't get carried away. I have kept this exclusionary bedroom practice over the course of my 20-year marriage—and most nights, I sleep like a baby.

Lastly, make sure you do not drink caffeine (chemical stimulation) or alcohol (interrupts deep and dream sleep cycles), do work (mental stimulation), or exercise (physical stimulation) within three hours of going to bed—as each of these can interfere with getting a good night's sleep. Set yourself up for sleeping success and you might just find you have a better outlook in the morning!

WHAT'S WITH ALL THE YAWNING?

Yawning is an involuntary action in which we open our mouths wide and inhale. And even though yawns are involuntary, everyone knows that they can be quite contagious. They are thought to be related to fatigue, tiredness, or boredom, but the actual reason behind why we yawn continues to elude scientific researchers. So we continue to guess that it must have to do with taking in more oxygen in order to put us into a somewhat more wakeful state. By the way, while I was writing this I felt compelled to yawn about seven different times—just to check it out!

To Nap or Not to Nap...

How come naps can be really wonderful some days, and others you wake up in such a fog, it seems it takes you an hour just to shake it off?

Well, it all has to do with timing. If you think back to the architecture of sleep, you'll recall that it takes about 90 minutes to pass through one complete sleep cycle. So if you were to lie down for a one-hour nap you would be waking up right about at the point where deep sleep begins. That would be the reason your brain is all woozy and your body is dragging around the house in search of another pillow. The best prescription for nap taking is to either devote a full 90 minutes to it or to settle for a 15-to-20 minute catnap, which avoids the deep sleep stages of sleep altogether. If you are having difficulty falling asleep at night, however, I suggest you forgo the nap and save up your "sleepy tokens" for nighttime use.

Rest, Relaxation, and Recreation

"Busyness is next to godliness" could be our nation's motto. When we get together with friends (or even with complete strangers) we can be found comparing schedules. Why are we so impressed by breakneck busyness and compelled to jam one more activity into an already full day? All work and no play make Jack a...*sick boy*. Aside from actual sleep, your body needs other forms of downtime to be truly healthy. This comes in three related forms: rest, relaxation, and recreation.

Rest is best thought of as a break time that is inserted into your busy day. It is a time of refreshing ease, inactivity, or tranquility that takes place after a period of exertion or labor. I like to call them "Sabbath moments." Teatime, feet up, flipping through a magazine for 5 to 10 minutes, or sitting on the porch sipping a cool drink while watching birds fly by—that sort of thing. Yet we need an even greater period of uninterrupted rest each week. After building the entire universe, our God put aside one day in seven to rest. Who are we to think we can work straight through the week, pausing only to attend church, and not have to pay the piper in some way?

Relaxation is a more prolonged period of time spent avoiding bodily or mental work or effort. It is purposeful pleasure-seeking. Book-reading, hammock-swinging, taking a long walk—these relaxing activities refresh the mind and soul. Devoting 30 to 60 minutes to these activities in periods peppered throughout your week will go a long way in providing your body and mind with a powerful stress reliever.

Recreation. Dissect that word and you'll find it provides an opportunity for "re-creation." Recreation is the refreshment of one's mind or body that comes through activities that amuse or stimulate us. Adults grow up, and often we forget to take time to play, laugh, and have some old-fashioned fun now and again. So take up a sport, rent a comedy, go on a vacation, or if finances are tight, go on a "day-cation"...anything. Just cut loose and cut up (joke around). Studies have confirmed that often it is during these times when your mind is in neutral that you gain insight into difficult problems, achieve sudden solutions, or gain new insight that you were lacking during times of intense effort.

So do yourself a favor—add to your schedule some protected times when you can simply kick back and get yourself some rest, relaxation, and recreation. You will be blessed if you would just rest.

● ● ●

Not much more needs to be said in this chapter, except maybe, "Good night." I'll see you in the morning—bright eyed and bushy-tailed. Sweet dreams!

NEHEMIAH'S WAY OF PUTTING IT ALL TOGETHER

STEP 1: Cry out to the Lord

STEP 2: Seek His forgiveness

STEP 3: Ask for His empowerment for success

> **Prayer:** *Dear Lord Jesus, I never really knew all the wonders You created when You designed sleep. I am fully aware now that I have put my body at a great disadvantage by not getting enough sleep and rest. Please forgive me for wearing away at my health by neglecting this all-important area of rejuvenation. Lord, I ask that You would give me Your power to change my ways—and would You keep me as dedicated to protecting and preserving my well-being though proper rest and relaxation as I am at this very moment? In the name of Jesus I pray, Amen.*

STEP 4: Take an honest assessment of your health

1. On average I get _____ hours of sleep a night.

2. My pre-sleep habits (circle):

      Need major improvement   Could use some tweaking
      Are pretty good

3. I observe my Sabbath day rest (circle):

      Never   Occasionally   Sometimes   Frequently   Always

4. I schedule a rest period/work break into my daily schedule (circle):

      Never   Occasionally   Sometimes   Frequently   Always

5. I make time weekly for recreational fun (circle):

      Never   Occasionally   Sometimes   Frequently   Always

STEP 5: Verbalize your commitment to change

The person or group I will tell about my intent to improve my health in this area is: _____

STEP 6: Develop a detailed plan of action

I plan to make the following changes in my life with regard to sleep, rest, and recreation:

1.

2.

3.

4.

5.

STEP 7: Use the buddy system

Someone who may want to join me in making this better-health change (or who I could trust to keep me accountable) is: _____

5

Fueling Up for the Road Ahead

Filling Your Tank
with High-Octane Foods

Get up and eat, for the journey is too much for you.

1 KINGS 19:7

You've probably heard the saying "You are what you eat." When I was a child that always conjured up a funny vision of me walking around in a banana outfit, like on the old Chiquita banana commercials! But that saying holds so much truth. The more scientists research the components of foods, the more we understand that both health and sickness can be traced back to what we have fed ourselves.

Sadly, many in the church today are dying from self-inflicted wounds. We suffer from the same rates of heart disease, type 2 diabetes, and cancer as those outside the church—and even more disturbing is the fact that we have the world beat when it comes to obesity. (According to a recent study, Christians are more obese than non-Christians, and Baptists are in the lead.) Most of us live life overfed yet undernourished. It is time we separate from the world's eating patterns and instead strive to eat our way back to better health. Can I get an amen?

When you get right down to it, *food is basically fuel*. And similar to gasoline, there are both low-octane and high-octane varieties. Low-octane foods contain little nourishment (the term "empty calories" comes to mind), are quickly digested, and leave us both undernourished and under the weather. In contrast, food sources that fall into the high-octane category are slower to digest and will therefore give you a longer full-feeling time, along with a steadier energy level. These foods contain rich nutrients which God designed your body to run on. For those of you who understand a bit about automobiles you can attest to the fact that if you fill up your car with fuel that is of poorer grade than its manufacturer intended, your car will begin to run rough and eventually, you will cause some major damage to its engine. The same is true for your physical body. God provides us with high-grade food sources meant to recharge our batteries when we run low, yet we continue to eat low-grade foods, subsequently wreaking havoc in our heart, blood vessels, brain, and so on.

We need to become mindful of the fact that when we eat, we are not just refueling our bodies for the next few hours, but we are providing our temples with the building blocks it will use to repair itself for the future. If you and I desire to have sound health for the God-directed tasks that await us, we'll need to choose high-quality building materials today. This will require some investigation. *Antioxidants, complex carbohydrates, essential fatty acids, phytonutrients, fiber,* and the benefit of a *lower fat diet* are frequently topics in magazine articles or in the news media—but do you understand what all these components of a healthy diet are, and exactly why they are good for you?

Throughout this chapter you'll find definitions of the major components of the foods you eat and drink, and then explanations of how they impact your body (His temple)—in either a negative or positive way. There are some nutritionally power-packed foods you should open your gates to, which aid health and fight disease. On the other hand, there are some real duds that you should wall off or significantly limit when it comes to your diet. When you are finished reading through this chapter, I guarantee you will have a whole new reason to praise the Lord for His amazingly detailed creation.

ELEMENT #1: MACRONUTRIENTS

The majority of the food we eat would be categorized as *macronutrients*, meaning we need a relatively large (macro) amount of these to live. Adam and Eve dined regularly on these macronutrients in the Garden of Eden. Fruits, vegetables, grain, and nuts likely comprised the whole of their diet. Meat was not on the menu. In fact, the Bible tells us that the very first animal that was killed was done so by God to be used as a sin-covering, a set of clothing for the sin-soiled first man and woman. Animals were sacrificed from that point on only as an offering to the Lord (see Cain and Abel), as spilled lifeblood had a redemptive purpose. It wasn't until after the Flood that the Bible reports that meat, poultry, and fish were added to the mix. In Genesis 9:2-3 God says,

> The fear and dread of you will fall upon all the beasts
> of the earth and all the birds of the air, upon every
> creature that moves along the ground, and upon all the
> fish of the sea; they are given into your hands. Every-
> thing that lives and moves will be food for you. *Just as
> I gave you the green plants, I now give you everything.*

Am I suggesting that you become a vegetarian in order to get back to the way things were in the Garden? Not at all, because then I'd have to join you; and I have yet to meet a meat I didn't eat. I just found this "vegetarian Bible fact" very interesting. If you are a vegetarian or a vegan, fabulous—just make sure you follow the healthy food guidelines we are about to discuss, because I've known many overweight, undernourished non–meat eaters. Vegetarian does not necessarily equal healthy.

Okay, let's fast-forward to our present-day food choices—meat, fish, grains, legumes, fruits, vegetables, and so on. Regardless of the particular foods we eat, our diets are comprised of three main components: *protein*, *carbohydrates*, and *fats*. And while all of these building blocks contain calories, not all calorie sources are created equal. A calorie, most simply put, is a measure of energy packed into a gram (about a thirtieth of an ounce) of food. Proteins and carbohydrates both contain four calories of energy (fuel) per gram of food, whereas fats contain over twice that much at nine calories per gram. Furthermore, there are different variations within each of these three groups—some of which you need to erect walls against—things you shouldn't eat so much of, and others you should enthusiastically open your gates to—nutritionally dense foods to welcome with open arms.

Proteins: You've Either Got 'Em or You Don't

The first macronutrient your body needs to survive is protein. Dietary proteins can come from animal sources, such as meat, milk, eggs, and cheese, or from legumes (beans) and nuts. Our bodies use protein molecules in a myriad of ways, such as to repair muscles and skin and strengthen bones; they act as hormones, digestive enzymes, and antibodies that fight off diseases. Furthermore they provide transportation for such things as the oxygen that rides around in your blood. And these are just *some* of the important functions that proteins perform within the body.

Each protein is comprised of a select combination of 20 different amino acids (which are complex molecular structures). If you ever studied chemistry, the structure of just one amino acid should be enough to convince you that there is an Intelligent Designer out there. Twelve of these intricate amino acids can be assembled within our bodies, and are therefore—as far as diet is concerned—called *nonessential amino acids*. The other eight must be ingested, and so are termed *essential amino acids*, because it is *essential* that we get them from an outside source in order for our bodies to function properly.[1]

Everyday living depletes the body of its protein stores, and therefore we must continuously restock our supply cabinet with this vital food component. Overall, protein should make up 25 to 35 percent of your dietary intake. So exactly how much protein should you eat in a day? Well, that depends upon who you are. If you are a bodybuilder or another type of athlete, you are going to require more than the average adult simply because you need more protein to repair all that connective tissue wear and tear (muscles, bones, cartilage, ligaments, and so on).

That said, protein deficiency is typically not a problem in the United States. We tend to overindulge ourselves in protein—especially meat-based protein. Big steaks, large chicken breasts, thick-cut pork chops are staples. What happens if you eat too much protein? Well, the processing of all that extra protein taxes both your liver and your kidneys and can lead to problems down the road.[2] Also, eating large amounts of animal proteins (meat and eggs) is one of the known factors that increase your chance of developing kidney stones. (You may want to rethink a high-protein diet. At the least, run it by a medical doctor or nutritionist for guidelines.)

When looking to fulfill your daily intake of protein, think about *quality* and *quantity*. As you'll see by reading through the list below, the lower the protein's saturated fat content, the better it is for you—we'll talk about this further in the section on fats. As for what a healthy meat-based protein portion looks like, you'll find some useful guidelines in the next chapter.

Lean, Healthy Proteins (Install "gates" here)
White meat poultry (skinless)
Pork tenderloin
Lean beef (10 percent fat or less)
Eggs
Low-fat cheese
Fish
Nuts, nut butters, seeds
Beans (legume-type, not string beans)
Yogurt
Low-fat milk (1 percent, skim)
Soy (soy milk, tofu, soybeans)

"Chubby" Proteins (Erect "walls" here)
Dark meat poultry (with skin on)
Sausage meats, hot dogs, and cold cuts such as salami and bologna
Beef (15 to 25 percent fat)
Whole milk, cream, half-and-half
Full-fat cheeses
Butter

RULES FOR STEADY FUELING

#1   Eat a good breakfast. (This rekindles your metabolism's "fire.")

#2   Have a healthy snack mid-morning and mid-afternoon.
      (This keeps your hunger down and your energy level up.)

#3   Stay well-hydrated.

#4   Limit caffeine intake (less than three to four cups per day).

#5   Eat to match your day's activity level.

#6   If you are still hungry after a meal, take seconds of a colorful
      vegetable—leave the meat, pasta, and potatoes alone.

#7   Don't eat while you are busy doing something else—you will
      typically overeat when your attention is elsewhere.

Carbohydrates: From Simple to Complex

The second macronutrient which needs to be a part of your menu is carbohydrates. All carbohydrates (carbs) are made up of sugar molecules. Carbs are the easiest food sources for your stomach to digest and as a result, they provide the most rapid supply of fuel for your body (in the form of pure glucose—the most basic form of sugar). How many times when you felt your energy level going south have you reached for a sugar or bread-based snack? Your body knows just where to find a quick fix.

There are two naturally occurring types of carbs and one that is man-made. *Simple carbohydrates* common to our diet include table sugar (sucrose), fruit-based sugar (fructose), brewed beverage (for example, beer), sugar (maltose), and milk-based sugar (lactose). *Complex carbohydrates*, or starches such as bread, rice, pasta, and potatoes, are made up of sugar molecules that are linked together in a chainlike fashion (hence "complex"). Even some fruits and vegetables like apples, cherries, grapes, corn, carrots, and sweet peas contain high amounts of carbohydrates. In their natural state, most complex carbohydrates are loaded with fiber—which is a good thing.

Refined carbohydrates are a man-made subset of complex carbohydrates that digest as quickly as simple carbohydrates. Refined carbs are typically made from processed grain, which has been stripped of its bran and subsequently its fiber and nutrition by the "revolutionary" milling process which became common in the early 1900s. Another way of refining carbs is brought to us by the juice industry. Apple juice and orange juice straight up are some of the worst things you can drink, as they digest in an instant, skyrocketing your blood sugar (more about this in the following chapter). The more refined a carbohydrate is, or should I say the less untangled it is with its fiber, the quicker it can be broken down into single sugar molecules, like that of simple carbs. White rice and refined flour used in pastas and baked goods are other modern-day examples of not-so-good-for-you refined carbohydrates.

When I learned this truth the first thing I did was alter my family's dinner menu. I made only brown rice (instead of white), and I stopped serving Italian or French bread with dinner. I also switched all our pasta to varieties that were fiber-filled. It took *six weeks* before my oldest child recognized the change and asked, "Hey—how come we never have bread with dinner anymore?" So I figured it wasn't that big a loss to them. I just made sure there were plenty of other things to fill up their bellies and excite their taste buds at meal times. Nowadays refined breads are a rarity in my home—almost as appreciated as a homemade cake!

STEALTH SUGARS HIDDEN IN YOUR FOOD

When we eat prepared or packaged foods, sometimes we get more than we bargain for…a whole lotta sugar, that is! Here is a list of foods that can sneak by you and sabotage your best efforts to cut back on the sweet stuff.

One Serving of...	Amount	Grams of Sugar	Approximate Teaspoons of Sugar
Table sugar (for reference)	1 tsp	4	1
Yogurt	single container	27	7
Applesauce	½ cup	25-27	6-7

One Serving of...	Amount	Grams of Sugar	Approximate Teaspoons of Sugar
Low-fat salad dressing	2 Tbs	8	2
Dried cranberries	1/3 cup	26	6.5
Granola bar	one	12	3
Ketchup	1 Tbs	4	1
Pickle chips (bread and butter style)	6 chips	6	1.5
Cereal	1 cup	24-40	10
Instant oatmeal (flavored)	1 packet	12	3
Spaghetti sauce (jarred)	½ cup	10	2.5
Peanut butter	2 Tbs	4	1
Tomato soup (canned)	1 cup	24	6
Coffee creamers	1 Tbs	6	1.5
1 percent milk	8 oz	12	3
Sports "waters"	8 oz	14	3.5
Orange juice	8 oz	22	5.5
Apple juice	8 oz	28	7
Grape juice	8 oz	39	10
Soda (one can)	12 oz	41	10

Carbohydrates need to be eaten in specific proportion to fat and protein. What that exact ratio is depends on who you're talking to; but the general consensus is that carbs should make up somewhere between 40 to 50 percent of your food intake each day.

What happens if you overload on carbs—like after finishing that huge New York-sized bagel or bountiful bowl of pasta? Well, because carbs digest so easily, your body is rapidly supplied with a huge load of fuel, most likely beyond what you currently need (unless you are about to go out running or something). When faced with this fuel overload, your body must store away this extra fuel in your fat, liver, and muscle cells for possible future use. Therefore a diet which is too high in carbs will lead directly to belly fat (among other locations), and eventually to a problem known as insulin resistance (a literal disease-maker)—which

I realize is a new term for many of you. Hold the thought for now; we'll talk about that subject in the next chapter.

Below are two lists to aid you in making healthier carbohydrate choices throughout your day. As a rule of thumb, the less processing a food undergoes (the more it looks the way that God created it), the better it is for you. The more fiber a carbohydrate food contains, the slower it will digest, and the longer you feel full after having eaten it. We can make sure we are building better "temple structures" by erecting walls against refined carbohydrates and installing gates that allow our bodies access to complex carbs.

Carbohydrates That Are Better to Avoid or Limit Significantly (Erect walls here)

White bread: sliced, bagels, Italian bread, dinner rolls, biscuits, hot-dog and hamburger rolls
White rice
White, Yukon gold, red potatoes
White pasta: all shapes and sizes, including noodles
White sugar…really, *all* sugar needs to be limited
Fruit juice
Soft drinks
Beer, wine, and liquors

Healthier Carbohydrate Options (Install gates here)

Whole-grain breads
Brown rice
Sweet potatoes
Whole-grain or low-glycemic-index pasta (such as Dreamfields brand)
Honey
Whole fruit instead of its juice (for example, apples, oranges)
Fruit juice diluted with 4 parts sparkling water (a great soft-drink substitute)

Fats: They're Not All Bad

Fat has gotten really bad press. It has gained a reputation as an evil foodstuff that must be purged from our diets. Yet God created this third macronutrient to fill a number of vital, life-giving roles. Fats are used by the body to make hormones, store fat-soluble vitamins (see below), and make essential fatty acids, which help to regulate your blood pressure and strengthen your immune system—to mention just a few of the good deeds it does around your temple grounds.

Fat is also a rich fuel source (remember, each gram yields nine calories of energy when compared to protein's and carbohydrates' four). Therefore weight gain is easily the result of overeating from this caloric-rich food category. This is the likely motive behind all the hysteria—and the reason why it is so important to limit dietary fat to just 15 to 30 percent of your food intake. But please don't shy away from *all* fats.

There are two primary types of fats: saturated and unsaturated fats. *Saturated fats* are typically solid at room temperature, and most originate from animal sources (meat, eggs, dairy). Most saturated fats are bad for your health *when eaten in large amounts* as they lead to elevated cholesterol levels and cardiovascular complications, among other diseases (see chapter 6). *Unsaturated fats,* which originate primarily from plant sources, are usually liquid at room temperature (with the exception of coconut and palm oil). As a rule of thumb, fats that are solid at room temperature are worse for you than those that are liquid. However, there are some saturated fats which are full of healthy nutrients (such as eggs and avocados), which when eaten in moderation are health-producing, rather than health-robbing.

The ultimate bad-for-you fat, which you should wall off ASAP, is *trans fat.* Found readily in manufactured snack foods (chips, crackers, cookies) and at your local drive-thru restaurant, these fats have been linked to heart disease. The evidence against trans fats is so damaging that California has just banned them being used in all food establishments across the Golden State. The Golden State—good; golden, trans-fat-cooked French fries—not so good!

Fats to Leave or Limit Greatly (Erect walls here)
Butter
Lard (for example, Crisco)
Whole milk and cheese
Cream, half-and-half

Fats to Love, But Not Overeat (Install gates here)
Olive oil
Canola oil
Flaxseed oil
Fish oil (omega-3's—see page 80)
Nuts (almonds, walnuts, pistachios)
Avocados—one of my personal favorites

Proteins, carbohydrates, and fats come in both low- and high-octane varieties. If you consistently choose better food options than the ones you are choosing now, you will not only have more energy, but you will suffer from fewer sicknesses, likely lose excess weight, and prevent the occurrence of many life-depleting or life-ending diseases.

If you are wondering if *I* ever eat from the lists of walled-off foods—of course I do. But I eat them sparingly, like condiments, and much less frequently than I do all those wonderful, good-for-me "gate" foods. I don't forbid myself a particular food, because that would only make me crave it (funny how human nature is—like Adam and Eve, we want the one thing we can't have). I simply keep these not-so-good-for-me foods to a minimum, and when I do indulge myself with a high-caloric treat (for example, fried chicken or ice cream), I help my body burn off some of those excess calories by getting active within the next two hours—before my body has a chance to store them away in my fat cells. In this case, if you use it, you won't "gain it." (A healthy body takes upwards of two hours to complete the job of pulling all that excess fuel out of circulation and stashing it away. So try to expend some extra energy while those digested food molecules are still floating around in your bloodstream.)

MEAL PLAN SAMPLER

Proteins, carbs, and fats; bad-for-you vs. better-for-you...So how do you take all that useful information and apply it to your food shopping list and meal preparation? Not to worry—below you will find a week of mealtime menu suggestions from my book *Diabetes: Are You at Risk?* These are meals I frequently prepare when cooking for myself, or for my family. Eat them in good health!

Day of the week	Breakfast	Lunch	Dinner
Sunday	High fiber, low sugar cereal, 1 percent milk, ½ cup blueberries	Tuna salad with chopped celery, peppers, onion, dressed with lemon juice and olive oil, salt and pepper, or light mayonnaise, served over a bed of salad greens	Baked chicken, brown rice with low-fat gravy (use sparingly), and steamed carrots
Monday	1 slice whole-grain toast (buttered lightly with butter/canola oil spread), 1-2 scrambled eggs	Black bean soup with chopped tomatoes, cilantro, lime juice, and a dollop of low-fat sour cream	Low-glycemic pasta with tomato sauce and meatballs (lean beef or pork and beef mix)
Tuesday	Steel-cut oatmeal topped with low-fat milk, walnuts, cinnamon, and a bit of brown sugar	Chef salad topped with ham, chopped hard-cooked egg, tomatoes, and a bit of blue cheese (a little goes a long way in flavor)	Homemade chicken and vegetable soup, one high-fiber or low-glycemic dinner roll
Wednesday	Egg-white omelet with diced tomatoes and low-fat cheese, turkey bacon	Turkey sandwich (1/2 or whole), low-fat Swiss cheese, mustard	Lean beef burger (no bun), tomato salad, grilled zucchini

Day of the week	Breakfast	Lunch	Dinner
Thursday	Low-fat cottage cheese, ½ banana, sliced almonds, drizzle of honey	Ham and cheese between two romaine lettuce leaves (instead of bread), carrot sticks with dip	Pork roast, cauliflower, broccoli and carrot medley, packaged brown-rice pilaf
Friday	Fried eggs (in olive oil), Canadian bacon	Tomato soup (made with 1 percent milk), ½ melted-cheese sandwich (for example, reduced-fat cheddar or Swiss)	Specialty chicken sausage (for example, with broccoli rabe and roasted tomatoes), baked sweet potato, broccoli
Saturday	Yogurt (low sugar), chopped strawberries, ¼ cup granola	Cold chicken breast meat, sliced tomatoes, low-glycemic pasta salad	Turkey chili topped with low-fat, shredded cheddar cheese

ELEMENT #2: MICRONUTRIENTS

In contrast to the large amount of macronutrients our bodies use in the form of proteins, carbohydrates, and fats, *micronutrients* are nutritional dietary elements our bodies require in much smaller (micro) amounts. Yet, however small the amounts may be, micronutrients are still vital to our health and well-being. The absence of any of these important nutrients from our diets can lead to terrible consequences, and in extreme cases, can even lead to death. The saying "Don't sweat the small stuff" does not apply here!

Vitamins and Minerals A to Z

I have spent over a decade reminding my children to take their vitamins. Now that they are teenagers, they have finally begun to take health matters into their own hands...now if I could just get my husband to remember to take his! Vitamins are so important, because without them food could not be properly digested, nor could your metabolism be properly regulated. Vitamins are also important components in a well-running immune system. Quite simply, vitamins are biological *co-enzymes* (or "helper catalysts") whose very presence enables chemical reactions (such as digestion) to take place—similar to the role that yeast plays in the process of fermentation that causes bread to rise. Without a necessary supply of vitamins, the God-designed processes within our bodies will fail.

There are two groups of vitamins that our bodies require, fat-soluble and water-soluble. *Fat-soluble vitamins* A, D, E and K can be stored in the body's fat and liver cells, and therefore need replacement only every few days. *Water-soluble vitamins*, namely C and the B-complex (B1, B2, B3, B5, B6, B12), are flushed from the body in 1 to 4 days and must be continually replenished. An entire chapter could be written on all the benefits vitamins afford our body, but for the "Cliff Notes version," use the chart below as a quick reference guide.

Vitamin	Area of Effect in the Body[3,4]	Best Food Source[3,4]
A	Eyes, bones, skin	Green and yellow vegetables
B1 (thiamine)	Metabolism, nerves	Egg yolks, whole grains, beans (legumes), fish
B2 (riboflavin)	Red blood cells, immune system, growth, respiration	Nuts, meat, cheese, eggs
B3 (niacin)	Circulation, skin, nerves, digestion	Meat, yeast, broccoli, eggs
B5 (pantothenic acid)	Hormones, immune system, metabolism	Beef, eggs, nuts, beans (legumes)

Vitamin	Area of Effect in the Body[3,4]	Best Food Source[3,4]
B6 (pyridoxine)	Cardiovascular, digestive, and immune systems, mental health	Egg yolk, wheat germ
B12	Blood (prevents anemia)	Liver, milk, eggs, fish, soy products
C	Tissue growth and repair, adrenal glands, gums, immune system	Berries, citrus fruits, green vegetables
D	Aids absorption of calcium and phosphorus (minerals), bones, teeth	Fish oils, dairy, eggs
E	Circulation, nerves	Cold-pressed olive oil, leafy green vegetables, beans, almonds, whole grains
K	Blood clotting, bones, metabolism, liver	Egg yolks, leafy greens, broccoli, cauliflower, cabbage

Minerals, another micronutrient essential for health, are naturally occurring elements found in the earth. Like vitamins they function as co-enzymes. Needed in even smaller amounts than vitamins, they are vital for proper functioning of our bodies. We require numerous essential minerals such as *iron,* which helps to transport oxygen in the blood, *calcium,* which is vital for the formation of strong bones and teeth, and *zinc,* which plays significant roles in metabolism, immunity, cell growth and division, wound healing, skin and eye health—even in your sense of smell and taste.

Deficiencies in essential minerals can lead to all sorts of health problems, as you can imagine. So make sure your diet (at best) or your multivitamin (at least) contains the current recommended amounts of these essential elements. (The USDA recommendations do change from time to time. Most vitamin and mineral supplements will tell you on the label how much of the Recommended Daily Allowance (RDA) of each micronutrient it contains.)

Antioxidants Fight Free Radicals

Much has been said about the micronutrient *antioxidants* lately. And while most people know they are something good to include in their diet, many don't have any idea as to what they are and how they work—because nobody ever explains *that* part. So let me begin by first introducing you to some of these antioxidants—namely vitamins A, C, and E. Antioxidants such as these protect healthy cells from damage caused by unstable molecules known as *free radicals.*[5] A free radical, very simply put, is a chemically "needy" molecule that longs to be completed by a single oxygen molecule. The problem is that when it grabs that oxygen molecule from a healthy cell in the body, the cell is weakened or damaged as a result. Free radicals have been strongly linked to cancer, heart disease, and aging—so they are certainly not something you want roaming around your body.

Where do all these free radicals come from? Everyday digestion of foodstuffs yields a fresh batch of free radicals. This would be quite manageable if we didn't have behaviors that "super size" the free radical load within our bodies. When we digest high-fat meats, eat charbroiled delicacies, smoke tobacco, are under emotional stress, or even when we get badly sunburned, free radicals are created in abundance. The moral of the story…avoid burnt food, burnt skin, and burning tobacco—and make sure you get plenty of antioxidants every day. (Today there are literally thousands of antioxidants science has identified, and the latest research seems to show that the best way to get these antioxidants is from food sources rather than synthetic vitamins.[6])

TOP TEN ANTIOXIDANT POWER FOODS

#1   Small red beans

#2   Wild blueberries

#3   Red kidney beans

#4   Pinto beans

#5   Cultivated blueberries

#6   Cranberries

#7   Artichokes

#8   Blackberries

#9   Prunes

#10 Raspberries

American Chemical Society, "Largest USDA Study
of Food Antioxidants Reveals Best Sources," *ScienceDaily,* 17 June 2004.

The Colorful World of Phytonutrients

Now here is a nutritional gate that may be new to many of you. Phytonutrients are plant-based chemicals that, while not essential for life, have been shown to prevent many diseases, such as stroke, heart disease, cancer, and macular degeneration (a real vision stealer for many older people).[7] Many different phytonutrients have been identified, and I am sure we will continue to discover more in the future…God's creation is just that intricate.

These days food corporations take every opportunity to highlight the healthy components of their products, so those of you who are package and label readers may recognize some of these plant-based chemicals such as *carotenoids*, *luteins*, and *flavonoids*. They are found primarily in bright or deeply colored fruits and vegetables. Some of the best dietary sources of phytonutrients are *dark leafy greens* (broccoli, kale, collard, and spinach), *yellow and orange plant-based foods* (sweet potatoes, carrots, peaches, and apricots) and *red-fleshed fruits* (tomatoes, pink grapefruit, watermelon, and guava).

Many Americans eat less than the Center for Disease Control's recommended five servings of fruits and vegetables per day, and when they do, they often avoid the deeply colored, phytonutrient-packed options like those listed above. You wouldn't decorate for a party using all white, beige, and brown decorations—so don't decorate your plate that way either. Do yourself a tremendous favor and put some color onto your plate; it'll turn a boring meal into a fiesta of nutrition and flavor.

Omega-3 Fatty Acids

Cold-water fish offer us a rich source of omega-3 fatty acids, another of the micronutrients. Fatty acids are unsaturated fats (see above section on saturated vs. unsaturated fats) that are essential to your body's health. Omega-3 fatty acids play a crucial role in brain function as well as normal growth and development. They are considered essential because you are not able to make them on your own, and therefore it is critical that your diet provides them.

While there are omega-6 and omega-9 fatty acids also, most nutritional focus has been placed on omega-3's because they have been shown to decrease the chance of death from sudden cardiac arrest (heart attack) by 50 percent![8] Other added advantages to adequate omega-3 consumption include lowered cholesterol, triglycerides and blood pressure, decreased symptoms from arthritis, decreased osteoporosis, improved psychological wellness, decreased attention deficit disorder symptoms, decreased occurrence of breast, colon, and prostate cancers, and decreased macular degeneration.[9] If you happen not to be a fish-eater, you do not get a pass—see the list below for other options.

Foods high in omega-3 fatty acids:

Fish such as salmon, halibut, sardines, albacore and
    light chunk tuna, trout, herring, catfish, cod
Walnuts
Flaxseed and canola oil
Shrimp
Clams
Spinach

THE FINAL ELEMENTS: FIBER AND FLUIDS

Three Cheers for Fiber!

There is a running joke in my family—actually, my kids are responsible for it—that if a food item in my home is high in fiber then I must be the culprit. "Fiber is Mom's best friend" jokes abound. Sometimes, I must admit, I do go overboard…like the time I tried to get them to eat hamburgers (another rare treat) on these unappetizing "fiber buns," which I agree look like flattened hockey pucks. But seriously, anytime I can switch out a food staple with one that is higher in fiber (and not begin an outright revolt), I do.

So what's so fabulous about fiber, or *roughage* as our grandparents used to call it? Unlike the preceding foodstuff categories, fiber is not something that is digested or absorbed in our stomach or intestines. In other words, it doesn't provide us with any *nutritional* value.

Something else you may not know about fiber is that it exists in two forms: *insoluble fiber*, which does *not* dissolve in water and *soluble fiber*, which when dissolved in water becomes a gel-like substance. Basically insoluble fiber's claim to fame (not to be too graphic) is that it comes out in the same form in which it goes in—unaffected by our digestive enzymes. Because of its "tough" nature, it adds bulk to our stool and increases the speed at which our solid waste moves through our digestive system. The body's solid waste is filled with toxic chemicals, so the quicker we can move that stuff along and show it "the back door," the better we are health-wise. Soluble fiber, on the other hand, has been found to lower blood cholesterol and sugar (glucose) levels—a great benefit.[10]

The Mayo Clinic recommends a minimum of 20 to 30 grams of dietary fiber per day: 30 grams for men and 20 grams for women under age 50. As you age, your body needs even more fiber, so it is recommended that men and women over 50 increase their fiber intake to 38 and 25 grams respectively. Nutritional labeling is very helpful here when eating packaged or prepared foods. Below I've listed the most fiber-friendly whole foods you can eat so you can find creative ways to bulk up your diet.

High-Fiber Food Sources[11]			
(1 cup cooked portion unless otherwise noted)			
Legumes 13-16 grams/ serving	**Vegetables** 5-10 grams/ serving	**Grains** 4-7 grams/ serving	**Fruit** 4-8 grams/ serving
Split peas	Artichoke: 1 med.	Whole-wheat spaghetti	Raspberries
Lentils	Peas	Barley	Pear: 1 med.
Black beans	Broccoli	Bran flakes	Apple: 1 med.
Lima beans	Turnip greens	Oatmeal	Strawberries

Drink Up!

Keeping yourself well hydrated is as important to your temple as it is to your houseplants. That is because nearly 60 percent of your body's composition *is* water. Your body loses water each day through urine and stool, perspiration, and respiration. While 20 percent of your fluid intake should come from the food you eat (another reason to eat more fruits and vegetables) the other 80 percent requires that you drink approximately eight glasses of fluid daily. This way you'll be sure to replenish your body's own natural juices.

God made water to be the best source of hydration—zero calories, inexpensive, and refreshing. So while other fluids (juice, milk, alcoholic and caffeinated beverages) do count, they should really be kept to a minimum, as they contain too much extra baggage (calories, caffeine, and cost). And here's a tip: The next time you are hungry, drink a glass of water first. You'll find you eat less, and on some occasions, you may even realize that your thirst was masquerading as hunger—and you'll be able to save yourself some unnecessary calories.

Now for those of you who depend on a daily dosage of caffeine (like me)—great news! Research studies have found that drinking healthy caffeinated beverages will decrease your risk of type 2 diabetes by *20 percent* for tea drinkers (caffeinated black tea) and *25 percent* for coffee drinkers. But what if you drink decaffeinated coffee? Congratulations on making such a wise beverage choice. Your chance of getting diabetes is lowered by a whopping *33 percent.*[12]

Green tea is all the rage today—and for good reason. It has about one seventh the caffeine of black teas, and it is chock-full of antioxidants. A recently released study has shown that drinking just one cup of green tea a day lowers the risk of lung cancer *fivefold* in nonsmokers and *thirteenfold* in smokers—now that is incentivizing.[13] (Truly an important finding for everyone, as 20 percent of lung cancers occur in nonsmokers.) This past year I have begun the habit, on most days, of drinking one cup of green tea mid-morning in addition to my early morning and late afternoon black tea times. I don't thrill to the taste of green tea, but I know my body smiles when it sees it coming, so I follow through with my commitment to improve my health as far as it depends upon me.

● ● ●

That was a lot of important information to digest, wasn't it? To sum up, here's the way I view the whole "food as fuel" issue: If you eat well the majority of the time, then a little "party food" here and there is a harmless treat. God created food for our nourishment and obviously for our pleasure. Typically, the closer foods look to the way God originally made them, the better they are for us. So eat whole foods (unrefined) and foods "in the raw" (uncooked) more often. Your body will thank you, as you will be laying a firm foundation for your future health—all for the purpose of strengthening and prolonging your service…for heaven's sake!

NEHEMIAH'S WAY OF PUTTING IT ALL TOGETHER

STEP 1: Cry out to the Lord

STEP 2: Seek His forgiveness

STEP 3: Ask for His empowerment for success

> **Prayer:** *Dear Lord Jesus, I am so thankful that You created food as a fuel source and as a pleasure to be enjoyed—in moderation. Yet I confess that I have not been feeding my body wisely. I was designed to function best when fueled with wholesome, natural food sources, just as You created them to be.*
>
> *Please produce in me a desire to eat life-giving foods, and help me to stop craving foods that would harm my health. Give me control—power through the Holy Spirit—to love myself as You love me and evidence that by the foods I choose to eat. May the food I place in my mouth be an act of worship to You. I am determined to fuel my body well so I can serve You with vigor until the day You call me home. In the name of Jesus, I pray, Amen.*

STEP 4: Take an honest assessment of your health

1. I eat a healthy breakfast (circle):

   Never Occasionally Sometimes Frequently Always

2. I eat a healthy mid-morning and mid-day snack to curb my hunger (circle):

   Never Occasionally Sometimes Frequently Always

3. I have an adequate source of vitamins and minerals in my diet (food or supplement-based) (circle):

   Yes   No

4. Do you have a good source of omega-3 fatty acids in your diet (food or supplement-based)? (circle):

   Yes   No

5. On average, I consume _____ servings of fruit and vegetables each day.

6. I drink 6 to 8 glasses of water (8-ounce) per day (circle):

   Never   Occasionally   Sometimes   Frequently   Always

7. I tend to eat more simple carbs than complex carbs:

   Yes   No

8. I tend to eat more saturated proteins (beef, dark-meat poultry) than lean proteins:

   Yes   No

9. I tend to eat more saturated fats (whole milk, butter, and cheeses) than unsaturated ones:

   Yes   No

10. The "bad for me" food indulgences I need to initially re-move from my diet and then add back in as an occasional pleasure (when I can maintain better control) are:

   _____

   _____

   _____

   _____

   _____

STEP 5: Verbalize your commitment to change

The person to whom I will verbalize my intent to improve my health in this area is: _____

STEP 6: Develop a detailed plan of action

I plan to add the following power-packed foods to my diet:

1.
2.
3.
4.
5.

I plan to significantly limit the following food or drink items:

1.
2.
3.
4.
5.

I will be sure to have these foods available to have as my healthy snacks:

1.
2.
3.
4.

STEP 7: Use the buddy system

Someone who would want to join me in making this better-health change (or who I could trust to keep me accountable) is:

_____

Waist Not, Want Not
Weight Loss That Stays Lost!

Whether you eat or drink or whatever you
do, do it all for the glory of God.

1 CORINTHIANS 10:31

M y mom's side of the family was Sicilian. Family get-togethers were always centered on the food. Not only were hours spent shopping and preparing for the meals, but a typical extended-family "eating frenzy" would last throughout much of the day. A common phrase heard around our dinner table was "mangia"—*eat!* With every ladle of food served, the underlying message seemed to be that love was being ladled out as well. Food somehow became a tangible form of love for us.

I was taught that the entire eating experience was one to be savored and prolonged. For example, whenever one of our multigenerational, multicourse meals was finally "finito" (finished), the men would sit around the table playing card games amid the crumbs while the women cleaned up the dishes. Yet even before the table was fully cleared, bowls of assorted nuts and fruits were brought out to munch on...as if we had not just consumed enough calories for days to come. When a couple of hours had passed and people were just able to re-button their pants, round three—which included pastries, cake, espresso, and after-dinner liqueurs—would begin, and the eating frenzy would resume... along with everyone complaining about how full they were. Yet each of us still somehow managed to make room for dessert.

The biblical term for eating more than you need is *gluttony*. In Ezekiel 16:49, God lists the sins of Sodom: "pride, *gluttony*, and laziness" (NLT). He doesn't even recount their sexual corruption; rather, gluttony gets billed as one of the top three sins that lead the Lord to dramatically obliterate the entire city of Sodom. Consistently eating too much is something to confess, repent of, and then turn from. God graciously makes it clear to us that overeating is a sin because, as with all other unholy acts, He wants to save us from becoming trapped in a yet another health-sapping, kingdom-weakening lifestyle.

The approach to weight loss I present here is not an uphill battle, but rather a steady push forward—completely doable and maintainable for the rest of your life. It's a way to *live*, not *diet*. The information you'll gain here, if applied, will change your life and the lives of those you come in contact with, forever—because frankly, what you don't know *can* kill you.

How Fat Grows

Everyone realizes that if you eat too much and move too little you will eventually gain weight, right? But how come fat seems to pile up on some people faster than others? Genetics does play a significant role, because each individual is born with a predetermined number of fat cells their body can fill. However, the body does have another opportunity to make extra fat cells. This occurs during late childhood through pre-adolescence; and the number of extra fat cells made at this crucial time depends on a person's body mass. Therefore, obese youngsters will generate more fats cells during this phase than lean ones. After that, most people's fat-cell count is set (with the exception of the extremely obese, as fat cells which are "filled to the brink" have been shown to divide[1]).

The filling of fat cells, though, is determined primarily by how many extra calories you consume throughout your day—because *everything you eat must be either used or stored*. Food digestion triggers your pancreas to regulate the upcoming rise in blood-sugar level by releasing the hormone insulin. Insulin restores blood-sugar balance by promptly packing away any extra calories into your body's fat, muscle, and liver cells. Any unneeded calorie source—carbs, proteins, or fats—will be broken down and stored away within your body's fat cells.

Another problem with chronic overeating or poor diet choices (high sugar, refined carbs) is that it leads to consistently higher levels of insulin circulating in your blood. The greater the level of insulin, the more your body will be driven to store digested calories away as fat. So if you have a history of eating too much (or too much of the wrong foods) you will be plagued with the problem of putting on weight more easily than others. That is how you've trained your metabolism to work.

Now let's approach this weight issue head-on. First we must accurately determine how much of you there is before we discuss what needs doing. So grab a scale, a soft tape measure, and a calculator.

Body Mass Index (BMI)

Most people play a guessing game when trying to figure out if they need to lose weight and if so, exactly how much. A better way to approach this decision is to find out how much you *should* weigh. The *body mass index* (or *BMI*) is a helpful tool that shows you the weight range that you should be shooting for. This scientific measurement takes into account both your height and weight and then categorizes you into one of four groups: *underweight, normal, overweight,* or *obese* (see the chart below). BMI results are valid for most individuals, with the exception of the elderly (less-than-average muscle mass) and the muscular athlete (higher-than-average muscle mass).

There are two ways to figure out your BMI. The easiest way is to go to my website, www.LisaMorrone.com, and click on Free Resources/ BMI Calculator. Simply enter your height (in feet and inches) and your current weight (you do need to get on the scale) and hit the "Find BMI" button. Instantly you will see, in full color display, in which category your weight places you, along with an explanation of your associated health risk. This free resource also gives you the ability to insert alternate weight measurements until you find out exactly how many pounds you should weigh in order for you to be safely within the normal range again.

The second way to determine your BMI is with the do-it-yourself method. Grab a pen and a calculator and work through the equation below (remember to use inches and pounds, not centimeters or kilos). Compare your results to the chart below.

BMI Calculation

$$BMI = \frac{(\text{Weight in pounds}) \times 703}{(\text{Height in inches}) \times (\text{Height in inches})}$$

BMI*	Weight status
Below 18.5	Underweight
18.5—24.9	Normal
25.0—29.9	Overweight
30.0 and above	Obese

You'll notice that the BMI method does not have separate charts for men and women, or for body-structure type (petite or large frame), hence the need for ranges.

Body Type—Which Fruit Are You?

Have you ever heard health practitioners using terms from the produce aisle to refer to people's body types? I find this to be a clever and memorable way to typecast people. An *apple* figure describes someone who carries their excess weight around their midline (stomach, sides, and back). A *banana* body is long and lean, and has great *a-peel*! (Most people would trade their body type in for this model.) The third body type is the *pear*-shaped frame: A person who carries their extra "junk" in their hips and "trunk," or backside. So why is it important to know which fruit you are? Because research has found that those who are apple-shaped carry a much higher risk of disease and premature death than their pear-shaped friends. And bananas are much healthier than both apples and pears—*figure*-atively speaking.

Now an important word to my "apple buddies": The medical

community has issued stern warnings to people whose waist measurement (body circumference measured at the height of your belly button) is considered excessive. Below you'll find the waist circumference level *above which very high health risks* are experienced. If your midsection has placed you at high risk, on the following pages you'll find out what you can do about it.

Excessive Waist Circumference Measurements:

Men: at or above **40 inches** (101cm)
Women: at or above **35 inches** (89cm)

Waist-to-Hip Ratio

Doctors have discovered another important measurement for predicting a person's health risk, namely the *Waist-to-Hip Ratio (WHR)*. Studies have shown it to be a better indicator of type 2 diabetes in men than the BMI.[2] And still other research has found it to be a more accurate measure of obesity in the elderly population (since, as mentioned before, the BMI can be inaccurate here).[3]

The WHR is a quick test to perform on yourself—and the math equation is much easier. Simply divide your waist circumference (from the previous section) by the circumference of your hips, and the result will be your WHR. For the second half of this equation, wrap a cloth tape measure around the broadest point of your "hips" (or pelvis to us physical therapists). Remember to begin and end at the exact same point. If you run out of tape, mark your skin where it ends and pick up where you left off.

Now plug both your hip and waist measurement (in inches) into the equation below. Then look at the chart below and see where it lands you: *low*, *moderate*, or *high risk*.

WHR = Waist circumference ÷ hip circumference

Here is an example: If your waist circumference = *40 inches* and your hip circumference = *38 inches*, then your waist-to-hip ratio = 40 ÷ 38, or *1.05.* For some of you this simple home exercise will be an immediate wake-up call. Don't just hit the snooze button and go back to sleep. Take action now.

Waist-to-Hip Ratio Chart		
Male	**Female**	**Health Risk Based Solely on WHR**
0.95 or below	0.80 or below	Low risk
0.96 to 1.0	0.81 to 0.85	Moderate risk
1.0+	0.85+	High risk

What's So Bad About Being Overweight?

Up till now I have not dealt with the particular health issues that stalk people who carry excess weight. Now it's time to spell it out. If this seems frightening, you're right—it is. But just like we should maintain a healthy fear of God, we also need to have a healthy fear of lifestyle-related disease. If any of the diseases or disabilities listed below happens to become your disease, you will no doubt be relegated to the sidelines of God's Super Bowl game.

- type 2 diabetes
- heart disease
- stroke
- high blood pressure
- osteoarthritis of weight-bearing joints (hips, knees, foot and ankle)
- cancer (breast, colon, and endometrial)
- dementia
- obstructive sleep apnea
- gallbladder disease
- fatty liver disease
- gout

- varicose veins
- abdominal hernias

For a more detailed discussion of these ailments, pick up a copy of one of my earlier books: *Overcoming Overeating* or *Diabetes: Are You at Risk?*

How to Become a Real Loser

In 2004 a very popular television program, *The Biggest Loser*, debuted. Season after season found contestants competing against each other to see who could lose the most weight by a certain date, motivated, of course, by a cash prize. I wonder if all those pounds that were shed in the name of the almighty dollar have stayed shed in the years that followed. If weight loss is done for temporal reasons, then results are usually temporary. Don't just become a *loser*—become a *real loser!* You can be motivated by a much higher reason and fueled by a much higher Power so that you will have sustainable results that earn you eternal kingdom riches.

Every women's or fitness magazine and diet book to hit the market seems to propose a "new" way to lose weight. Over *50 billion* dollars was spent last year in the United States alone on diet plans and books—making it one of our nation's largest industries. The fact is that most reputable diet plans will work—if you are able to stick to them. The problem is...most people can't.

Why is that? Well, that is the subject of my earlier book *Overcoming Overeating: It's Not What You Eat, It's What's Eating You!* I believe 75 percent of overeating is done for emotional reasons. If you begin any diet plan without first understanding (and healing from) *why* you are driven to eat too much, then even the best diet will not bring about lasting results. If this chapter is speaking directly to you, get a copy of that book for yourself—it will be transforming for your body, mind, and soul. After you have addressed the emotional aspect of your overeating, then you can learn new habits and make lifestyle changes that are scientifically proven to trim off the extra you. In the following pages you'll find out how.

Reset Your Insulin Receptors

Earlier I spoke about insulin and how its job is to store away excess food energy in your body's fat, liver and muscle cells. The way it does this is by acting as a "key" that unlocks the individual *insulin receptors* on those cells, clearing the way for calorie storage. This is how your body deals with all those extra calories you eat—when everything is functioning as it was designed. The problem with chronic overeating or even moderately eating foods that are refined (sugars without fiber and simple carbs) is that over time it deadens the response of your body's insulin receptors to its own insulin.

You've seen something similar to this play out in the mall, I'm sure. If a small child calls once for his mom, her head whips quickly around to respond. However, if that child starts into a "Mommy, Mommy, Mommy" litany, then the mother's ears seem to become unable to pick up that frequency! When your blood teems with sugar (glucose), your pancreas naturally responds by releasing an overabundance of insulin that begins a "Store me, store me, store me" rant…and the request just falls on deaf ears. The result of *insulin resistance* is type 2 diabetes, belly fat, and cardiovascular disease—to name the top three.

Rein In Your Sugar Highs

The best way to resensitize your insulin receptors is by placing them on a sugar-spike fast. Basically the goal is to give your pancreas a rest and your insulin receptors a chance to reset their sensitivity. You do this by following the first two weeks of an eating plan (such as the South Beach plan) that strictly limits foods that cause rapid rises in your blood sugar. You limit your food intake to moderately sized portions of lean proteins, low-fat dairy, eggs, and vegetables—but no high-sugar veggies such as corn, peas, beets, or carrots. Cardiologist Arthur Agatston (author of *The South Beach Diet* book) reports that two weeks on such food restriction resets your body's insulin sensitivity and positively affects blood chemistry levels (fats, sugars, insulin). For more details, I do recommend his book, as I have personally witnessed those results play out a dozen times in friends, family members, and my patients— along with significant weight loss.

SNACKS THAT STEADY YOUR BLOOD SUGAR

The best way to keep your blood sugar steady, and your food cravings at bay, is to take care not to let your sugar levels drop too low. A below-normal blood sugar level will most certainly send you on a "carb hunt," looking for a quick energy boost between meals. And even if you are able to fight off those cravings, you will likely show up at your next meal ravenous and eat many more calories than you should. My patients frequently ask me what *I* eat when I get hungry between meals. Well, I have certain favorite "go-to" snacks that I eat mid-morning and again in the mid-afternoon. Most times I grab one of the following:

- Half an avocado, teaspoon of blue cheese dressing, black pepper
- A handful of almonds or walnuts
- Approximately 25 pistachios
- A low-fat cheese stick
- A carrot, apple, or half a banana with a tablespoon of peanut, almond, or cashew butter
- A small Greek-style yogurt (low sugar/high in protein), topped with cinnamon
- Low-fat cottage cheese with honey and cinnamon, topped with berries or banana slices
- Hummus with cucumber or sweet pepper slices, or 5-6 baked, multigrain pita chips
- A small piece of dark chocolate
- A mini bag of microwave popcorn (no trans fats), sprayed with a misting of olive oil

And remember, everyone needs to be allowed to eat a cookie or a handful of chips occasionally—I am not suggesting an inflexible approach to life.

Reboot Your Muscles

The second scientifically proven way to resensitize your insulin receptors is with physical exercise. Studies have found this result to occur time and time again, although they still don't understand *how* it works. The standard recommendation is to become physically active—walk the dog, rake the leaves, wash the car, clean the house, bike, swim… whatever! Just try for 30 minutes of movement three to five times a week. Not only is it good for your body, moderate exercise improves mental outlook and strengthens your immune system while you're at it.

Maximize Your Metabolism

Another aspect of becoming a "real loser" is to make sure that you take advantage of the way in which God designed your metabolism to work most efficiently. In order to get a handle on this, think of your body's metabolism as a campfire. When you rise in the morning, your metabolism's "fire" has burned down to hot coals. In order to start it burning again you must begin by adding small kindling. When larger flames begin to catch hold you can add bigger sticks and eventually, good-sized logs to that fire. Once a steady blaze is achieved, your fire will have no trouble igniting and incinerating whatever is placed on it (within reason). You'll need to tend to the campfire of your own metabolism in much the same way. The key is to keep your body's fuel (food) supply from running too high or too low throughout the day. Let me share with you three things you can do to keep your metabolism burning efficiently with a steady supply of "firewood."

The Breakfast of Champions

God designed our bodies to survive the night without food, but in the morning we are supposed to break that fast with breakfast. The number-one problem with sluggish metabolisms is that they never get stoked in the morning. A cup of coffee and a piece of dry toast just won't do it. Or worse yet is not eating anything until two hours after you've gotten up from bed. Eating late in the morning is like dumping an armload of logs onto smoldering coals…not much chance of them catching fire!

You need to get in the habit of eating a balanced *meal* of slowly digestible foods for breakfast. Some of you may protest, *But I'm just not hungry in the morning.* Yet here's the thing—if you don't give your body some nourishment right off the bat, the rest of the day will be downhill from there. First of all, by mid-morning you will be so hungry, and your blood sugar will be so low, that your body will crave a quickly digestible carb—like a bagel or muffin. Your blood sugar will shoot up after eating that, your pancreas will crank out a huge load of insulin in response, and then your blood sugar will fall below normal again—often within the next hour or so. And guess what? Yep, you're hungry again. The best breakfast contains protein and a complex carb—just as we spoke of in the last chapter.

Food Combos That Slow Digestion

The best way to keep your blood sugar steady is to feed your body food combinations that make your stomach work longer at the digestion process. (Remember, quick digestion leads to skyrocketing blood sugar.) A fabulous suggestion proposed by authors Grossman and Hart (a physician and a dietician, respectively) in their book *The Insulin-Resistant Diet*[4] is that whenever you eat, you include a protein source. Another great idea they offer is to partner equal servings of proteins with carbs, such as eating an egg with a slice of whole grain toast. Both of these methods have the excellent effects of slowing digestion and keeping you feeling full for much longer.

Personally, I've been using these eating guidelines since I first learned of them two years ago, and I can tell you that my fasting glucose level, my cholesterol level and ratios, and my body weight have all improved as a result. And it is so much easier than I thought—I simply adjusted what I bought at the market to make sure that I had a variety of healthy (and tasty) protein sources on hand, like different nuts, avocados, reduced-fat cheese, and high-protein Greek yogurt.

Finally (and you're going to love this one), get into the habit of having a bit of butter or a dip of olive oil with your bread. According to Dr. Agatston, the very presence of that fat (even a bad-for-you fat like pure butter) has a positive effect on your blood sugar, as it slows the digestion of the carbohydrate you are eating along with it.[5]

Power Snacking

Another crucial thing you must do to lose pounds (or to remain slim) is to snack. The name of the game is to keep your blood-sugar levels as even as possible, for two reasons. First, it will help to eliminate high sugar spikes, which trigger fat storage. Secondly, it will keep your hunger in check so you are not in "starvation mode" by the time your next meal rolls around.

So in between meals, when your blood sugar begins to dip, you need to respond by adding a log onto your "metabolic fire" in the form of a healthy snack. I suggest you plan ahead for these mid-morning and mid-afternoon snacks by having some of the appropriate foods I've mentioned before on hand, such as low-sugar/high-protein yogurts (Greek style is the best), nuts such as almonds, walnuts, pecans, or cashews, avocados, low-fat cheese sticks, carrot sticks with peanut butter, and so on. If you work outside the home, remember that portability is an important factor. Healthy snacks have to be easy and easily accessible if they are to work for you.

Scale Back

I was speaking with a pastor from Ghana, Africa, the other day. He told me that his weight has "ballooned" after coming to live in the United States. His downfall, he said, is that unlike Ghana, food in this country is everywhere! Boy, I couldn't agree with him more. We are a super-sized, oversupplied nation when it comes to food. Unfortunately, most of that food is in our stomachs one moment and entering our bloodstream as sugar the next. Even though there is food aplenty available to us, we do need to keep in mind that we don't have to eat it all.

Portion Control

In *Overcoming Overeating*, I discussed the issue of what a normal-sized portion looks like.[6] I am not the type to weigh and measure my foods, but if that works for you—have at it. For us others, we can try to keep these visual helps in mind:

A serving size of...	Is about the size of...
meat or fish	your palm, and about as thick as your index finger

A serving size of...	Is about the size of...
lean fat (cheese)	a one-inch square cube
carbs (rice, potatoes)	a scoop the size of a tennis ball
vegetables	the insides of your two cupped hands
fruit	your fist

It is also helpful to use packaging information to make sure you know exactly what constitutes "one serving size." And do yourself a huge favor—don't eat out of containers, packages, or cooking pots. You'll always overeat. Also, stick with first helpings only unless you are headed back for more fresh veggies.

HOW TO CONTROL YOUR EATING WHEN YOU'RE AWAY FROM HOME

Calories add up whether you eat them at home or away. Some of the biggest food traps are found in restaurants, at the home of a friend or family member, or when you're on the road traveling for business or pleasure. In each of these situations you'll face similar challenges—you're not the chef, someone else is serving you, food is more abundant, and it is harder to say no when the food is extra special or your host is extra nice. So here are some tips to help you keep your portions healthy—no matter where you graze:

When dining in a restaurant

1. Don't choose an all-you-can-eat establishment...who needs all that temptation anyway?

2. Send the bread basket back. If you love bread (or are famished), take a small piece of bread with some butter or better yet, olive oil, and then send the rest of it away. (Adding the fat here in moderation satisfies your hunger and controls your blood sugar better than bread alone.)

3. Eat only half of your meal and "doggy bag" the rest. (If you don't have the will power to stop halfway through, ask your waiter to package half of it before you begin.)

4. Order an appetizer and a salad instead of an entree.

5. Share a dessert if you absolutely must indulge.

When sitting down to a meal with friends or family

1. When someone initially invites you over for dinner, casually mention your healthy eating goals so that he or she can be aware of and accommodate appropriate food choices for you, if possible. For example, you could say:

   - "I'm watching what I eat right now, so don't feel pressure to prepare a feast for me."

   - "I've been avoiding rich foods lately, so could I contribute by bringing the vegetables or salad to the party?"

2. Don't go hungry. Eat a hunger-satisfying, protein snack before arriving.

3. In conversation before the meal, make a gentle reference to your new health goal of reining in your food portions.

4. When served something that looks great, but is not great for you, compliment the chef on its aroma and appetizing look. But, maintain your healthy perspective by being positive and say something like, "I'll have to bend my food rules today so that I can enjoy a taste of this amazing dish!" (Then take a small portion.)

When traveling

1. Don't go empty-handed. Think ahead and pack some high-powered foods for the car or plane. For my family this is nuts, fruit, low-fat cheese sticks, balanced nutrition bars, and plenty of water.

2. Make any fast-food stops where you know they offer lean proteins, vegetables and salads, and fruits.

3. Don't allow yourself to get hungry…snack between meals so that you are not tempted to overorder and overeat.

Choose Better Food

Exercise your right to vote when it comes to what you will eat. Life is all about choices, and food choices, good or bad, are made one at a time. Try asking yourself these questions the next time you reach for something to put into your mouth: Does this food benefit my temple? Does it look like something God has created (a whole food, not heavily processed)? Will it strengthen my ability to serve Him in the long run? Would I be proud of fueling my body this way if Jesus was sharing this meal or snack with me? If you are starting to have doubts, chances are you can find yourself something better to eat.

Rich Foods Can Make You Poor

My husband's mother cooks up an amazing feast each year for Thanksgiving Day. Yet her recipes always make me chuckle. If the instructions call for butter, she uses extra; if it says to add half-and-half, she'll use heavy cream. My mother-in-law thinks the way most Americans do: the richer the food, the yummier it must be. Not to mention that we all fall prey to indulging ourselves around holidays.

The fact is that we live in very affluent times. Food in the United States is still relatively cheap when compared to the rest of the world. But just because we can afford to buy rich-type foods, and just because they are in plentiful supply, doesn't mean we should load up on them. We will have all eternity to dig into amazingly rich food when we are seated around the banquet table of Christ. Let's choose to eat a bit more "poorly" in this life so we can live longer and serve Him stronger down here.

Empty Calories That Fill You Up

Pastries, cakes, and basically anything white (cauliflower *not* included) will fill your stomach without adding to your nutritional wellness. These lackluster foods are like throwing paper on a roaring fire. Sure, they cause a big, bright flare-up at first, but almost as quickly as the blaze began, it dies down. In other words, it has no staying power. Make the most of each bite of food. Be diligent to find nutritionally dense alternatives such as lean proteins, legumes (beans), colorful vegetables, and high-fiber fruits (apples, nectarines, and so on). This way not only will you be filled up and satisfied, you'll also be fueled up and sanctified!

Quenching Your Thirst Without Expanding Your Waist

Do you know how many extra calories soft drinks, 2 percent or whole milk, and fruit juices can add? Hundreds, thousands, and tens of thousands throughout the year! Drinking just one can of soda or 12-ounce glass of orange juice a day (150 to 165 calories each) can pile upwards of 15 to 17 pounds on in one year's time. Yes, orange juice has vitamin C in it—but that doesn't mean you should drink it in large quantities. God created the orange as a whole fruit (juice *with* fiber). And as far as I can tell, there weren't any juice bars in Eden.

I always tell people, "Don't waste your calories on drinks." Water straight up, or with a twist of lime or lemon, is a staple at my home, as is sparkling water with a splash of fruit juice. In fact, I've convinced my kids that one part orange, grape, pomegranate, or cranberry juice mixed with three parts sparkling water *is* soda. Try it out in your own home, and let me know if you begin to see your waist shrinking.

Put Some Muscle into It

Want to supercharge your weight-loss efforts? Then you must increase the number of calories you burn each day. Muscles are much hungrier than fat. They eat up far more calories each day just "living." So the more muscle you can build, the faster you'll burn off calories you've ingested. And when we use those muscles, it is like adding flammable liquid to our metabolic fires, as calorie requirements rise sharply and even stay elevated for about an hour or so after you slow down. So even while you are cooling down, your calories are burning up.

Building Bigger Muscles

Our muscle strength diminishes as we age (picking up speed after passing our fortieth, "over-the-hill" birthday). Deliberately calling on those muscles to "get off their bones and do something" is the only way to build them back up. Now that I am in my forties, I see that my leg muscles (which used to be quite athletic) have begun to deflate. And strength training is where I have found my temple maintenance routine could use the most attention. It is also the part of my health maintenance "program" which is, quite honestly, lacking the most. This is why I refer to health as a journey, not a destination. None of us will ever quite arrive at perfection this side of heaven...yet we must stay in hot pursuit of wellness if we are to be of use to God down the road.

"Use it or lose it" definitely outlines the problem. Muscles will grow larger only if they are taxed with loads that are beyond what normal living places on them. So muscle mass is predictably increased by lifting weights, exercising (or performing tasks that require strength and vigor), or by lifting the weight of our own bodies against gravity (Pilates-type exercise is an example of this). The best approach, if you have the time, is to systematically strength-train your skeletal muscles. Building up your body's largest muscles (for example, your thigh and buttock muscles) will have the greatest impact on your metabolism. For those of you who don't have a whole lot of time to dedicate to a strength-training circuit, I will show you some key muscle-building exercises in chapter 8 that are quick and simple enough for anyone to add to their daily routine—even me!

Get a Move On

It is a simple principle—the more you move, the more calories you'll burn. Muscles, heart, and lungs that are working harder require more food in the form of calories. The more intense your workout is, the more food calories you will burn through to fuel your activity. In the chart below you'll find examples of typical forms of exercise and the approximate number of calories they burn. As noted, the actual numbers of calories burned will depend not only on the activity you choose, but also upon your body weight. A larger body will require more caloric energy to keep moving. (Seeing this chart in black-and-white can make eating those two 100-calorie cookies not worth all the effort it takes to burn them off!)

Activity / Calories burned during 30 minutes of exercise[7]	Body Weight			
	120 lbs	140 lbs	160 lbs	180 lbs
Aerobics	222	258	294	333
Basketball	225	264	300	339

Activity / Calories burned during 30 minutes of exercise[7]	Body Weight			
	120 lbs	140 lbs	160 lbs	180 lbs
Cycling (10 mph)	165	192	219	246
Golf (pulling clubs)	138	162	186	210
Hiking	135	156	180	201
Jogging	279	324	372	417
Skating (ice and roller)	177	207	237	264
Skiing (snow and water)	171	198	228	255
Swimming (moderate pace)	239	270	309	348
Tennis	180	207	237	267
Walking	195	228	261	291
Weight training	198	228	261	294

● ● ●

God has gifted you with the potential for good health. As part of your stewardship of His temple-gift you have the opportunity and the reason to restore and maintain your body weight within a "normal" BMI range. The information we've covered here will supply you with all the construction materials you need to pour a solid foundation on which to build better health for your tomorrow…for His kingdom's sake.

NEHEMIAH'S WAY OF PUTTING IT ALL TOGETHER

STEP 1: Cry out to the Lord

STEP 2: Seek His forgiveness

STEP 3: Ask for His empowerment for success

> **Prayer:** *Dear Lord Jesus, I now understand that being overweight has put my life in great jeopardy. I ask for Your forgiveness for the way I have been using food to fill up my free time and to manage my negative emotions—instead of asking You to fill my empty feelings and to heal me. Please be my power source to overcome this habit of misusing food. I want to dedicate my weight loss plan to You, for Your glory. May everything that I refrain from putting in my mouth be a sacrifice of praise to You. I want to be a better representation of a person who has all their needs met in Christ alone. In the name of Jesus, I pray, Amen.*

STEP 4: Take an honest assessment of your health

1. My BMI calculation (if needed, see BMI calculator at www.LisaMorrone.com) places me in this category (circle):

   Underweight   Normal   Overweight   Obese

2. My risk factor for disease as predicted by my WHR is (circle):

   Low   Moderate   High

3. When I combine my BMI with my waist circumference, my associated health risk is (circle):

   Unaffected   Increased   High

   Very High   Extremely High

4. I presently suffer from these possible weight-related disabilities or diseases (circle):

>Osteoarthritis (*knees, hips, ankles, low back*)

>High blood pressure   High cholesterol   Type 2 diabetes

>Cancer (*breast, colon, endometrial*)   Obstructive sleep apnea

5. I need to lose _____ pounds in order to get myself into the "normal" BMI category.

6. I need to lose _____ inches from my waist to become "low risk" according to the WHR predictions.

STEP 5: Verbalize your commitment to change

The person to whom I will verbalize my intent to improve my health in this area is: _____

STEP 6: Develop a detailed plan of action

I plan to make the following steps toward weight reduction and maintenance:

1.

2.

3.

4.

5.

STEP 7: Use the buddy system

Someone who would want to join me in making this better-health change (or who I could trust to keep me accountable) is:

_____

7

Line Up Your Spine
Postures That Preserve Good Health

He holds victory in store for the upright.

PROVERBS 2:7

Sunday mornings on my way into church I often stop to hug a dear older lady, Becky, who always arrives ahead of me, all set to worship her Lord with song. Her eyes still sparkle with life—but Becky's *body*...well, that's a different story. She'd be the first to tell you that it gave out long before she was ready to retire from serving the Lord. At least three different times Becky has told me how heartbroken she is to have had to give up her nursery duty on Sunday mornings—all because her neck pain got so bad she could no longer lift the little ones. While her spirit is still willing, her temple became prematurely weak.

Many aches and pains begin with bad posture. Faulty posture places excessive, harmful stress on the joints, discs, and muscles surrounding your spine. This pressure can cause early degenerative changes such as arthritis and disc bulging or herniations. What began simply as bad posture can leave you living in a temple filled with pain. Physical pain prohibits way too many Christians from carrying out God's ordained tasks. They have no other option but to minimize their involvement in kingdom work.

The material that follows is taken from the chapter about posture in my first book, *Overcoming Back and Neck Pain*. It is, hands-down, the book's most popular chapter. I have received dozens of e-mails and personal accounts of how simply changing a particular posture cured people's chronic back or neck pain. One woman reported that her neck pain of five years resolved "miraculously" overnight. Another person with a three-month ordeal with sciatica had this to say:

> My back has been hurting for 3-plus months—throughout this period of time I have had low back pain, upper back pain, knee pain, tail bone pain, and terrible sciatica at times [pain running down the leg]—my pain kept growing and getting worse and worse. Each morning I have had to stand at the kitchen counter in order to read my Bible because I just couldn't sit down—my sciatic pain was so awful. Seeking relief I've spent $600 on acupuncture, $300 on chiropractor work, both of which helped—but only temporarily.

> Then I picked up your book last weekend, read a couple of chapters, and came to the chapter about posture (sleeping, standing, sitting, and so on). Well, all I did was turn my pillow the other way—the one under my knees—and two days later (today) I woke up a new woman! I'm serious. I'm blown away. I could put on socks and tennis shoes without any pain—typically this sends pain straight down the back of my leg, AND I could sit down with my coffee and have my quiet time with the Lord!

This woman told me that she was ready to resign from her leadership role in ministry because she couldn't even sit long enough to read her Bible. Time and time again, people are truly amazed by the results they experience. I am not. As a physical therapist I have been teaching postural correction for over 20 years. I have seen thousands of patients, friends, and family members helped and healed by implementing healthier postures throughout both their days and nights.

This posture chapter even captured the attention of Pat Robertson's international television broadcast, *The 700 Club*. In 2008 I was asked to come on their Wednesday show, which is dedicated to health topics, in order to teach their television viewers the ways and means of lining up their spines. So I'm not going to mess with its success. In keeping with Nehemiah's rebuilding theme, this chapter will provide you with clear directions as to how you can effectively wall off destructive postures and instead install sound postural gates (correct postures) that will protect your body from deterioration and ease the physical pain you may be experiencing.

● ● ●

When Solomon chose to use the word *upright* in Proverbs 2:7 (above) he was likely not referring to posture—rather to an admirable personality trait equated with honesty, integrity, and being right with God. The word *upright* can also be used interchangeably with the word *integrity*, which can be further defined as "an unimpaired condition; soundness." If we apply that second idea of "upright" to the human body, a person whose spine is no longer upright has lost his or her structural integrity. Simply, their body is no longer sound and stable. And if I can take some license here with this verse: Physical victory over pain and disability can be in store for you if you live life in a more naturally upright position.

Good posture is all about regaining and maintaining a sound, stable, unimpaired position. All of the structures in our backs and necks (bones, discs, ligaments, nerves, and muscles) function best when they are upright, or well lined up. Poorly aligned posture is the culprit behind many painful back and neck conditions. It can be responsible for the development of muscle tightness, arthritis, disc disease, and ligament laxity. By learning the components of good posture, you can have your spine function optimally and avoid needless pain and injury—not to mention all the down time and fruitless years that may result.

The Results of Poor Posture

Our bodies are designed with the ability to put up with a great many bad choices. However, when we make bad posture choices and then hold ourselves in them for long periods of time, we bring our body to the breaking point. Many of my patients ask me, "Well, how come, if I've always sat or stood this way, do I have pain *now?*" I like to use the analogy of a sponge when trying to answer this question. If you begin slowly adding water to a dry sponge, it's fully capable of absorbing that water. But, over time, the sponge fills up, reaching its full capacity. Any further addition of water, and the sponge will begin to overflow. That is analogous to our pain. When we reach the body's capacity to absorb any further insult or injury, we feel pain. Some of us just "fill up our sponges" more quickly than others—and bad posture is a major reason for this early filling.

So if you find yourself developing back or neck pain while you are sitting at the computer, driving your car, or trying to relax at home on the couch, then the key to your healing will be found in *how* you sit. Or, if you have pain after standing awhile, say in line at the store or on your feet at work, then your standing posture needs to be overhauled. If you wake after a full night's sleep and are greeted by Mr. Pain, I believe you can ensure a healthy night's sleep by learning how to align yourself properly.

Maintaining postures that are well lined up is crucial to your healing from present pain, preventing future pain, and preventing or stopping further damage to your spine's many components. Our moms must have somehow instinctively known this. This is why so many of us heard the mother-mantra "Stand up straight!" throughout our teenage years. Just as with the funny faces we made, Mom surmised that if we didn't stop doing what we were doing, we would "stay that way." And for many of us, that prediction has come true.

Just to drive the point home, improper posture over time leads to:

- muscle shortening
- muscle weakness and fatigue
- muscle spasms
- loss of range of motion in the spine, hip joints, and shoulder joints
- worst of all, arthritis and disc derangement (bulging or herniated discs)

That's a lot of bad stuff, right? (Now don't you wish you'd listened to your mother?)

How did we go from being a slump-shouldered teen to an adult with a bad back or neck? Let's visit the teenager whose mother is always badgering him about his posture. Today he is again slumped at the computer for an hour while instant-messaging his buddies. At this age his muscles, ligaments, and discs are still healthy.

Fast-forward ten years. The teenager's slumped posture has now resulted in *dysfunction*—the loss of flexibility and shortening of structures in the body. Now, because of the muscular shortening that has occurred, he *can't* just "sit up straight" even if he wants to. His pain is now classified as dysfunction-syndrome pain. He must first work on the dysfunctional (tight) structures by applying the appropriate muscle stretches found in chapter 8, "The 10-Minute Muscle Makeover." Only then will he be able to take full advantage of the posture corrections in this chapter. (In cases where stretching and postural corrections do not bring about pain relief, I do recommend that you seek professional medical treatment by a physical therapist or medical doctor.)

And given further time, chronically poor posture will cause the body to move beyond muscle tightness to muscle weakness, ligament laxity, and joint and disc breakdown.

Good Posture—Recovery from Pain

When considering posture, you'll find it helpful to view the body as a tower of blocks. First, you need a sturdy and well-placed base (bottom) block. In terms of the body, "block 1" is our feet and their placement relative to the rest of our "blocks." The second block to be properly stacked is the pelvis, or hip area. To be carefully placed above block 2 is block 3, the shoulders. Finally, we'll call the placement of our head and neck "block 4."

With blocks, the force of gravity will cause a badly aligned tower to tumble to the floor. The advantage our bodies have over a tower of blocks is our supporting muscles and ligaments. These structures prevent a poorly aligned body from collapsing to the floor. However, a badly aligned upright position comes at a high cost to our bodies—muscle spasms, joint wearing, or disc degeneration often result over time.

The remarkable thing about postural correction is that people can feel immediate relief with simple changes, regardless of which category their pain is in. Posture is unquestionably the linchpin of recovery from back and neck pain. That being said, I am in no way proposing that you *never* slump (as I am at times while typing this)—rather, that you spend *most* of your time well aligned. Then you can enjoy a good slump every now and then!

Sitting: Give Your Discs a Break

Much of our time is spent sitting. Often the *way* in which we sit has created pain for us. With this in mind, let's look at some sitting basics that are body-friendly.

Your Feet on the Floor

First, it is helpful to have your feet supported by the floor. Sitting with your feet unsupported increases the pressure inside your discs by 90 percent. This internal disc pressure is similar to the air pressure in your car's tires. The next thing you know, you have a bulge on the surface.

Your Back Arched

Second, whenever possible, you should have the base of your chair (the part you sit on) slope downward. This elevates your hips slightly above your knees, tipping your pelvis for-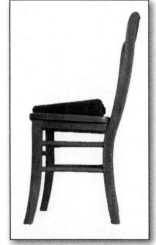ward and thus creating an effortless natural arch in your low back. This sloping can be achieved in a number of ways. If your car or office seat has an adjustable, angling seat base, take advantage of it. If not, you can buy a wedge-shaped cushion like the one pictured in figure 7.1. In a pinch, this wedge can also be made from a towel or even a folded pillow placed under your "buttock bones" (not your thighs).

This arched position of your low back (known as *lumbar lordosis*) can prevent the onset of 1) postural-syndrome pain, caused

figure 7.1

by the slumping of your spine to the point where its healthy structures begin to complain; 2) dysfunction-syndrome pain due to the stretching of shortened tissues; and 3) derangement-syndrome pain because of increased forces that slumping (or loss of your lordosis) has placed on your discs. Just one cushion, and all these bad boys can be sent away!

Is this "bottom up" setup always necessary? That depends on two things. Do you have pain in your back, neck, or head that is present or aggravated while sitting? Then yes. Do you sit for prolonged periods of time—for example, at a desk job or during the evening at the computer? Then yes, again. If, however, you are healthy and pain free and have a less-than-sedentary lifestyle with frequent position and postural changes, then this is not a must. Even if the latter is true, I do recommend you use the sloped position every now and then, especially when you know you'll be spending a lot of time seated (as during a long drive or when sitting through a long meeting or conference).*

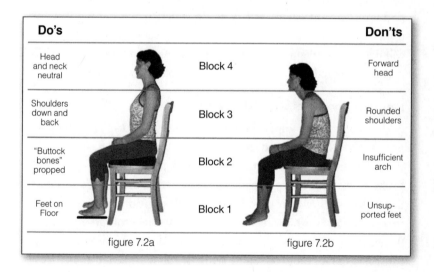

Do's		Don'ts
Head and neck neutral	Block 4	Forward head
Shoulders down and back	Block 3	Rounded shoulders
"Buttock bones" propped	Block 2	Insufficient arch
Feet on Floor	Block 1	Unsupported feet

figure 7.2a   figure 7.2b

---

* The only people I would not recommend this position for are those who have a diagnosis of *lumbar spinal stenosis*. In this condition there is narrowing of the bony tunnels (foramina) through which the spinal nerves (or possibly even the spinal cord) run. Creating an arch (lordosis) in the low back will further narrow these tunnels and may prove harmful. Those with spinal stenosis are more comfortable sitting with their low backs in either a flat or somewhat slumped position.

Do be aware that when it comes to creating a natural arch in your low back, you don't want to go to extremes. If your low back is too arched, you will be creating postural-syndrome pain or dysfunction-syndrome pain by going too far in the opposite direction. Moderately arched (neutral lordosis) positioning is best.

Shoulders: Down and Back

Now that you have your feet on the floor (block 1, figure 7.2a) and your thighs sloped downward so a low-back arch can be maintained effortlessly (block 2, figure 7.2a), let's move upward. As if constructing a block tower, you must next line up your shoulders (block 3, figure 7.2a) squarely over your hips. The way to get this block properly aligned is simple. First roll your shoulders up toward your ears, then back behind you, and finally, down toward the floor. Now hold them there. This "down and back" position of your shoulder block should feel fairly relaxed (though probably foreign). Not much effort should be required to maintain it. If you are experiencing pulling in your upper-chest muscles or where your neck meets your shoulders, you will need to supplement this postural correction with the upper trapezius and pectoral muscle stretches found in chapter 8.

Ears over Shoulders, Chin Slightly Tucked

Last—and most important for headache and neck-pain sufferers—is the position of your head and neck (block 4, figure 7.2a). While your shoulders are in the proper down-and-back position, draw your head backward so your ear opening lines up with the bony tip of your shoulder. When sliding your head back into this position, be sure you neither tip it backward nor tuck your chin way down toward your chest. When viewed from the side, your nose should be the prominent feature on your face (not your chin). Most of you will need to *slightly* tuck your chin (nod your head) to get yourself positioned correctly (see figures 7.3a and b).

Many years ago I had the pleasure of treating Emma, a lovely eighty-something lady. I say "lady" because she was poised, well-spoken, and gentle-natured. The reason she had come to physical therapy was neck pain. After an initial evaluation, during her first treatment I showed her a stretch to do at home. In addition, I taught her how to properly align her "blocks," with emphasis on blocks 3 and 4.

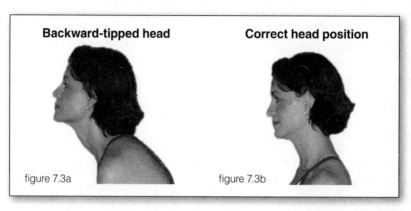

Backward-tipped head   **Correct head position**

figure 7.3a   figure 7.3b

When Emma returned for her next visit, she could barely contain her well-mannered self. As soon as she saw me she exclaimed, "I've grown! I've grown! Physical therapy has made me taller!" Surprised, I asked her to explain. She excitedly described how, when she'd gotten in her car to drive to therapy, she'd looked up into her rearview mirror. It was no longer properly positioned. So she slouched down into her "pre–physical therapy" posture, and sure enough, she could see into the mirror just fine. She readjusted her posture back to the new and improved position, adjusted her mirror to account for her "new height," backed out of her driveway, and smiled all the way to therapy.

Emma chuckled after telling me this and with a lively sparkle in her eyes said, "Who says you can't teach an old dog new tricks?" Proper posture most definitely changes the way you look, and apparently it changes your point of view too.

Guarding Neck Health

The alignment of your upper body (blocks 3 and 4) is essential to the health of your neck. It protects against arthritis and disc degeneration. When your shoulders are slumped forward, you must tip your head backward to maintain postural balance and keep your eyes looking straight ahead. This backward bending of your head creates a forward gliding of the lower neck bones and discs, which brings about two harmful results:

1. *An increased amount of weight borne on the facet joints of the neck.* This excessive weight-bearing can lead to arthritis or degenerative joint disease (DJD), which can eventually give rise to osteophytes and lateral stenosis.

2. *A wearing down of the spinal discs,* which, over time, leads to bulging or herniated discs and degenerative disc disease (DDD).

Pain resulting from DJD, lateral stenosis, or DDD can be felt directly over the area of the injury, or it can travel up the neck or down between the shoulder blades. It can even travel down the arms as far as the fingers.

My father-in-law has been diagnosed with lateral stenosis in his neck (narrowing of the bony passages for the spinal nerves of the neck). Formerly, every time he sat at the computer for any length of time, he would develop pain in his neck that would travel all the way down his right arm. The pain would get so intense, he would have to get up. Through analyzing his head and neck position, he realized that because he was having trouble reading the monitor, he would jut his head forward on his neck (leading with his chin) in order to get a closer view.

After having suffered horribly for months, he discovered he was able to avoid setting off his neck and arm pain simply by moving his monitor closer to his eyes and not the other way around. This way he could maintain his head (block 4) over his shoulders (block 3), all the while keeping a slight chin tuck. Did this postural correction cure his stenosis? Of course not, but it did allow him to protect the nerves in his neck from becoming compressed—and therefore it "cured" his posture-associated pain.

Another common effect of the slumped-shoulder-backward-bent-head posture is headaches. Most headaches of a mechanical nature are the result of shortened or compressed structures at the base of the head and dysfunction of the first few cervical (neck) joints. When the head is tipped backward, muscles at the back of the neck, along with the upper neck joints, become stiff and tightened. These shortened structures cause the nerves at the base of the skull to become compressed.

In turn, these tight muscles and inflamed nerves can produce headaches at the base of the skull, at the back and top of the head, and ultimately in the forehead. Headache and pressure that is sometimes felt behind the eyes can often originate from the upper neck area. If you suffer from headaches, from neck or back pain, or from radiating pain, numbness, or tingling in your arms or legs, then it is imperative that you give your head and neck posture an overhaul.

Standing: Realigning Your Body to Avoid Pain

Now let's turn our attention to standing posture. If I were to sneak up on you and take your picture while you were standing in the checkout line, which posture might best represent you? Are you putting your weight over your "favorite" leg (figure 7.4)? Have you lost the arch in your low back (figure 7.5)? Has your pelvis shifted forward over your feet so you are "hanging on your ligaments" (figure 7.6)? Where are your shoulders and head placed?

Standing posture is all about balance—the balancing of our weight over our feet (our base of support). When we are standing, our bodies are the most susceptible to the downward pull of the force of gravity and to side-to-side or front-to-back pushing forces. Gravitational force is a given, and there is no escaping it. The pushing (or shearing) forces our bodies must endure can come from outside the body (as when carrying a backpack over one shoulder or getting shoved at a crowded party) or inside the body (poorly aligned posture blocks). It is these horizontal forces that will eventually lead to the breakdown of our joints, ligaments, and discs. Further, when our blocks are not properly aligned, this also creates an undue amount of work for our postural muscles. Because they are overworked, these muscles go into spasm and create pain.

I have an experiment for you to try that will help you to feel this increased muscle activity for yourself. Stand up and place your fingertips along the vertical muscles of your low back (one to two inches away from your spine).

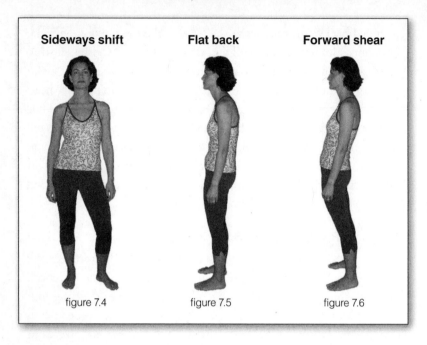

Sideways shift   **Flat back**   **Forward shear**

figure 7.4   figure 7.5   figure 7.6

First, tuck your chin and glide your head and neck backward to align your head block over your shoulder block. Feel the tone in your spinal muscles by gently pressing your finger pads into the muscle a few times. You should be able to feel a somewhat soft, springy muscle texture.

Next, jut your head and neck forward from your shoulders, leading with your chin. Again, push your finger pads into the spinal muscles. Now you will feel that the muscles are tense and don't give as you press into them. If you keep your fingers in place and move your head forward and back, in and out of good alignment, you should be able to feel the muscle tone increase as soon as you begin the forward glide of your head and decrease as you approach better alignment. Can you imagine how much work your low-back muscles have to do in order to hold up your forward-positioned head throughout the day?

A Firm Base of Support

With this in mind, let's go through the re-alignment of your standing posture from the ground up, just as we did with sitting. The base of support for standing is your feet. The optimal position of your feet is to have about four to six inches between them at the heels (figure 7.7). A stance in which your feet are placed closer than four inches together makes for a smaller base of support (figure 7.8). This causes your hip and back muscles to work overtime to keep you balanced. If your feet are spaced too far apart (figure 7.9), there will be subsequent injury to your knee joints and shortening of the outer hip muscle on both sides (the gluteus medius). These outer hip muscles are an important stabilizing force at the pelvis, and a wide-based foot position places them at a mechanical disadvantage. They will subsequently become weak and ineffective.

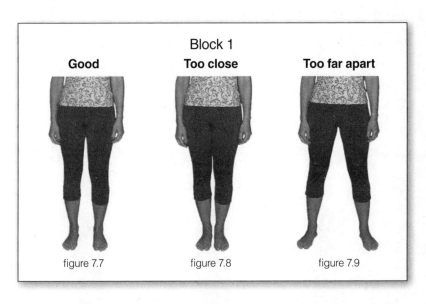

Block 1

Good	Too close	Too far apart

figure 7.7   figure 7.8   figure 7.9

Now that your feet are in the correct position, let's get your body weight equally balanced over them. You'll need to stand while reading this. First, rock your body weight over your right foot, then over your left, then back toward the center. Stop when you feel your weight is equally distributed over both feet. Next, rock or lean forward a bit (without bending your hips or knees) so you feel more weight on the balls of your feet (just behind your toes). Next rock your body backward, shifting your weight from the balls of your feet to your heels. Continue to rock forward and backward until you feel 50 percent of your weight on your heels and 50 percent on the balls of your feet. This may feel quite unnatural to you. But the proper alignment of block 1 is truly the foundation of good standing posture.

Years ago, correct standing posture felt very unnatural to me as well. When I first began attending college to study physical therapy, my standing posture closely resembled the one pictured in figure 7.11 (swayback). When my studies began to make me aware of all the physical side effects of my bad posture, I set out to retrain myself.

It was difficult at first. Every time I stood, I purposefully aligned my body. However, as my mind drifted off my posture and onto something else, I found myself reverting to my old ways. As soon as I noticed

Block 2

Flat back:	**Swayback:**	**Good back!**
• pelvis tucked • weight borne on heels • result: excessive disc pressure	• pelvis glided forward • weight borne on toes • result: excessive joint pressure	• pelvis aligned (with normal lordosis) • body's weight equally on heels and toes

figure 7.10   figure 7.11   figure 7.12

I was out of alignment, though, I would again reset myself. Over time, it became more of a habit, with less reminding necessary. A few months later, I realized that as soon as I slid back into my old posture, I felt uncomfortable. Now my body desired good alignment instead of bad. If you presently have pain (which I did not), your postural transformation will most likely be quicker than mine because *your pain* will remind you that your good posture has "left the building."

Your Center of Mass

The pelvis—block 2—is where our body's center of gravity (the middle of our mass) lies. It needs to be lined up over our ankles (actually, slightly in front of the ankle bones). We should have our pelvis tipped forward somewhat to create a low back arch (lordosis), as discussed earlier in this chapter. Proper alignment of the pelvis sets the stage for what happens with the shoulders, head, and neck.

Quit Slumping

Now on to block 3: your shoulders. This block needs to be aligned *over the pelvis,* not slumped as so many of us habitually carry ourselves (figure 7.13). The bony tip of your shoulders should be lined up with your hip bones when viewed from the side. Just like in sitting, the way you achieve this is to roll your shoulders first up toward your ears, then back behind you, then down toward the floor. The "down and back" position should be fairly relaxed, not requiring much effort to maintain (figure 7.14).

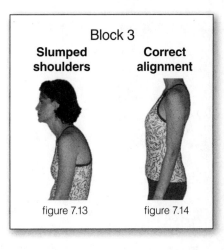

Everything in Line

Finally, we need to align block 4 (your head) over your shoulder block. The opening of your ears should be lined up with the bony tip of your shoulders (and following this line down through the hip and slightly in front of the ankle—see figure 7.15).

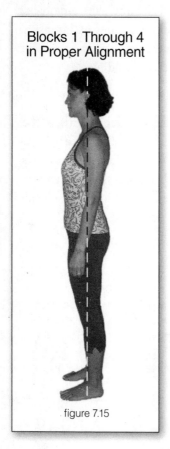

Blocks 1 Through 4 in Proper Alignment

figure 7.15

Getting your ear opening lined up with the tip of your shoulder is the first part of the proper block 4 position. Fine tuning is then achieved with the chin-tucked position (not a backward tip) of the head on the neck (go back to figure 7.3).

With proper alignment of these four blocks, your body will be a stable tower, able to properly bear the constant force of gravity. Sideways shearing forces will be minimized. Your joints, ligaments, discs, and muscles will be able to function in the way God created them to, optimally and with greatest mechanical advantage.

Though good standing posture often brings immediate relief from pain, that relief may be partial at first. After making these changes to their alignment, many of my patients report that their pain either decreases in intensity or that the amount of "real estate" it takes up on their body is diminished. In other patients, pain relief comes over time as posture corrections are supplemented with stretches or strengthening exercises. In either case, eventually your body will stop sending you those annoying pain telegrams and instead begin sending thank-you notes.

Sleeping: Don't Add Insult to Injury

If you have trouble getting comfortable at night or feel your worst when you get up in the morning, chances are you are not sleeping in an optimal position. If you suffer with arthritis, you are most likely very stiff in the morning. This is because your joints have been relatively immobile (still) all night. These postural changes will often bring dramatic improvement in your morning symptoms simply by placing your joints in less stressful positions during sleep.

First, sleeping posture is all about the pillows—how many you use and where you put them. So let's look at the three sleeping positions: *back-lying (supine), side-lying,* and *stomach-lying (prone).* Of these three, the first two are acceptable. Stomach sleeping is not good, however. (Before you stomach sleepers start protesting, let me tell you that I have a *modified* stomach-sleeping position that satisfies at least 75 percent of my patients who are just like you. Keep reading.)

On Your Back

Sleeping on your back needs only a few adjustments to make it a sound posture. Simply place one pillow under your *neck* and head (figure 7.16), not under your *shoulders* and head (figure 7.17).

Do...
* support your head and neck

Don't...
* support your shoulders
* Result: *your head will tip backward*

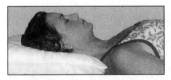

figure 7.16

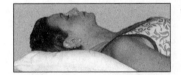

figure 7.17

Sleeping flat on your back with only one pillow under your head may not be an option for you if you have difficulty breathing or suffer from acid reflux or a hiatal hernia. These conditions do require an elevated head position. Usually someone with these concerns has two, maybe even three, pillows under their head at night, which puts their lower neck at significant risk for disc derangement.

Instead of this...

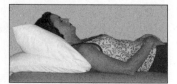

figure 7.18

Try this...

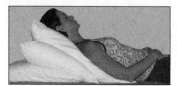

figure 7.19

If this describes your situation, you can use a modified "pillow pileup" that will protect your neck from injury caused by excessive forward bending. Figure 7.18 shows the typical pillow pile, in which all three pillows are placed perpendicular to the body. Figure 7.19 shows the first two pillows laid perpendicular, while the third (top) pillow is placed *parallel* with the body. This allows for elevation of the trunk, neck, and head rather than only the head and shoulders.

Some patients who sleep on their backs feel more comfortable with a pillow under their knees as well. When this is the case, I have found that people are even more comfortable if they simply change the pillow direction (figures 7.20 and 7.21). With the pillow turned lengthwise (parallel to the body), the entire thigh is supported, not just the knees.

From this...

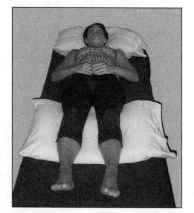

figure 7.20

Try this...

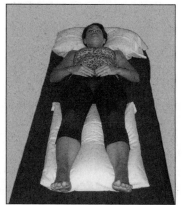

figure 7.21

On Your Side

Side lying is a great sleeping position as long as you have proper pillow placement. There needs to be enough support under your head to keep your nose in line with your breastbone (see figures 7.22 though 7.24).

Next, place a pillow lengthwise between your knees. This serves multiple purposes. It keeps your spine from rotating and side-bending (as your top leg drops toward the bed). It also prevents you from drawing your knees up toward your belly into a fetal position, if you are so inclined. (The fetal position is bad for the discs in your low back because it allows the internal disc gela-

Good head position

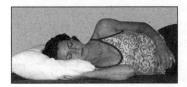

figure 7.22

Head too high

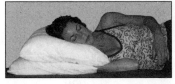

figure 7.23

Head too low

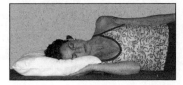

figure 7.24

tin to migrate backward toward your nerves). Lastly, a pillow between your legs helps to unload the weight of your top leg from the muscles of your spine (see figures 7.25 through 7.27).

The final pillow is optional for the person who suffers with low-back pain, but it's very important if you have neck pain or headaches. This pillow is placed lengthwise in front of your chest and abdomen. Its purpose is twofold:

- It relieves the pull of the weight of your arm and shoulder on your neck.

- It decreases rotation of the spine from below your neck, which creates a rotary stress on your lower neck. This in turn aggravates both your joints and your discs.

The pillow support between your knees and in front of your trunk can be achieved with a single four-foot-long body pillow (available at your local bedding and linen store). This way there are fewer pillows to keep track of.

On Your Stomach?

Now, it's time to address all you stomach sleepers out there. Let me explain why sleeping on your stomach is bad for your spinal health. In order to breathe in this position, you must turn your head fully to one side to clear the mattress or pillow with your nose. The discs in your neck and the joints of your spine are then held in that position for eight hours (or however long you sleep). This does not make your neck happy: 1) Your discs are structurally weakest when in the position of rotation, so this quickens their degenerative process. 2) Your neck joints don't like being held at end range. 3) The nerves in your neck are very sensitive to pressure and stretching. They don't like being twisted and held like that till morning.

The other parts of your body at stake are the discs in your low back. All discs receive their nutritional feeding primarily in non-weight-bearing, uncompressed positions, such as lying down. When you lie on your stomach, your

Good

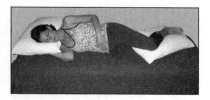

figure 7.25

Not so good

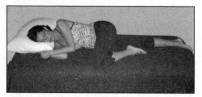

figure 7.26

Even worse

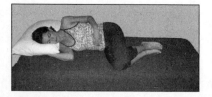

figure 7.27

spine is in a position of mild extension or backward bending. This creates compression of the back portions of the discs and the discs are unable to absorb nutrition in this state. Therefore, when you're sleeping on your stomach, the back portions of your discs do not get fed. No food = poor disc health, poor disc health = disc degeneration (DDD).

Pillow position for modified stomach sleeping

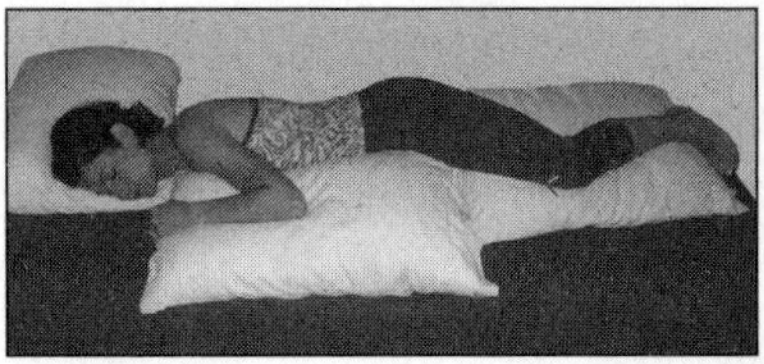

figure 7.28

So how can we remedy all this and still get a good night's sleep? Presenting… the *modified* stomach-sleeping position. Begin by setting yourself up as though you were going to sleep in the side-lying position described above. A body pillow works best here. The pillow under your head should be supporting your head only from your ear to the back so that your face is hanging off the edge (figure 7.28).

Now, turn your body toward the mattress, straightening your bottom leg. Your top leg and your trunk will be supported by the body pillow and your head will be rotated about 45 degrees toward the mattress, as opposed to 90 degrees when you're stomach-sleeping. This modified position gives you the *feeling* of full-front contact with your sleeping surface. Now you can sleep comfortably without stressing out your spine.

Six years ago I evaluated a physician's assistant who had been regularly referring patients to my office. She came in to see me herself one evening. She was having difficulty writing her patient notes because of severe fatigue and cramping in her right hand. She assumed it might be carpal tunnel syndrome (a compression of the nerves at the wrist). She wondered if I might be able to help her. She had a long history of neck pain with occasional pain spreading down into her right arm. She also reported disturbed sleep and waking each morning with numbness in both of her hands.

When I asked her what position she slept in—you guessed it—it was on her stomach. I enthusiastically explained my modified version. It was met with a less-than-enthusiastic response. "I've slept this way for over forty years. I don't think I'll be able to change." But she was a good sport (and motivated to get well), so she said she would give it a try.

When she returned for her first treatment session, she was a believer. Much to her surprise, she *was* able to get comfortable in this new position. Even more important, she wasn't waking with numb hands. With a combination of manual (hands-on) physical therapy and postural changes, she remains symptom-free to this day. (I know this because we became dear friends.) She does, on occasion, tell me, "I woke with numbs hands this morning. I found myself on my stomach. I must have lost my pillows during the night."

● ● ●

This patient and countless others like her continue to be living proof that these methods work. By paying attention to the positions we hold our bodies in, even as we sleep, we will find much healing can be had and much pain avoided. I know it to be true in my life as well as my patients' lives. So sit up, stand straight, eat your veggies, and have a good night's sleep—I'll see you in the morning.

NEHEMIAH'S WAY OF PUTTING IT ALL TOGETHER

STEP 1: Cry out to the Lord

STEP 2: Seek His forgiveness

STEP 3: Ask for His empowerment for success

Prayer: *Dear Lord Jesus, Wow, who would have thought that standing and sitting up straight was as good for my body as eating my vegetables! Forgive me for ignoring my mother (on both accounts) and for placing my body at risk with my often lazy approach to sitting and standing. From now on, as far as it depends on me, I want to protect my spine. Lord, would You prompt me both day and night to "line up my spine" for a healthier tomorrow? In the name of Jesus, I pray, Amen.*

STEP 4: Take an honest assessment of your health

1. I have back, neck, or limb pain that is:

   Nonexistent   Occasional

   Chronic/Bothersome   Limits my recreational activities

   Disabling/Interferes with my daily function

2. I slump when sitting (circle):

   Never Occasionally Sometimes Frequently Always

3. I slouch when standing (circle):

   Never Occasionally Sometimes Frequently Always

4. I sleep in one of the "better/best" positions shown in this chapter (circle):

   Never Occasionally Sometimes Frequently Always

5. I sleep on my *stomach* (circle):

Never   Occasionally   Sometimes   Frequently   Always

STEP 5: Verbalize your commitment to change

The person to whom I will verbalize my intent to improve my health in this area is: _____

STEP 6: Develop a detailed plan of action

I plan to make the following specific changes in my body's line-up with regard to my sitting, standing, and sleeping postures:

1.

2.

3.

4.

5.

STEP 7: Use the buddy system

Someone who would want to join me in making this better-health change (or who I could trust to keep me accountable) is:

_____

8

The 10-Minute
Muscle Makeover
Key Exercises to Improve
Strength and Flexibility

Wake up! Strengthen what remains and is about to die, for I
have not found your deeds complete in the sight of my God.

REVELATION 3:2

s a physical therapist, I've been treating the orthopedic problems
of my patients for over two decades. And let me tell you—
nothing breaks down a person's temple faster than muscle
problems. When God created our skeletons, He draped them with
muscles whose two primary responsibilities are to maintain our bodies in an upright posture and to act as the moving force that carries us
around in this world.

If your muscular system is neglected or underused, key "players"
will become stiffened or weak—sometimes both. When your temple's
musculature is left hanging in this precarious state for a long time, your
risk for physical injury or chronic disability mounts. In addition to
painful outcomes, deconditioned muscles run out of steam, fatiguing
earlier and earlier each day, it seems. If you feel as though you have to
drag yourself along just to get through the day, then this chapter will
be a real wake-up call for your sleepy muscles.

A few years back, I evaluated a patient who was having terrible hip pain. Carole was extremely frustrated because, besides the pain, she was beginning to put on weight since she was no longer able to participate in her weekly exercise classes. The pain even woke her up at night— each time she rolled onto the painful side. During my physical assessment I discovered a number of joint problems and muscle imbalances (tightness/weakness) in Carole's back, hip, and leg. At the end of that initial session there was just enough time left for me to teach her one exercise. I taught her a key hip-muscle stretch to begin at home.

Four days later when she returned for her first official treatment, she was all smiles. Carole reported that 70 percent of her hip pain was gone and she was no longer being awakened at night by pain. While my new patient was amazed, in all honesty, I was not. Her outcome was not unusual. An aptly chosen and consistently performed muscle exercise (or two or three) can have a profound healing effect. If today your body is feeling older than it should, and you find yourself lugging your "parts" from one end of your day to the other, why not give yourself a "muscle makeover"? What will take you only *ten minutes a day* will take years off your temple. In any economy, this makes for a wise investment.

Muscle Anatomy 101

The spectacular anatomy of skeletal muscles is one of the many evidences that an Intelligent Designer does indeed exist. It should come as no surprise that God has fashioned each muscle with great precision. On cross section each muscle resembles an electrical cable that itself is comprised of a bundle of other "cables," or *fascicles* (pronounced "FA-si-kuls"). Inside each of those fascicles is a grouping of linear "wires" which are actually the individual muscle cells (or fibers), all neatly aligned—running in the same direction—along the length of the muscle. (See figure 8.1.)

Each muscle cell (some of which can be up to two inches long) is made up of still smaller bundles of *myofibrils*. Zoom in even further with a high powered microscope and you'll see that each myofibril is made up of a series of contracting segments called *sarcomeres*. (See figure 8.2.) It is here, within the sarcomeres, that muscles actually do the work of contracting (shortening) or stretching (lengthening).

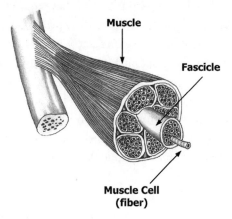

Muscle

Fascicle

Muscle Cell (fiber)

figure 8.1

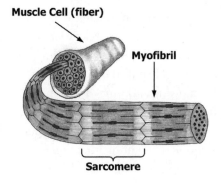

Muscle Cell (fiber)

Myofibril

Sarcomere

figure 8.2

Muscle Overload

Muscle injuries typically occur either because a muscle is *too weak*, or because it has become *too tight*. One way in which weakened muscles can become strained is when you attempt to lift or lower a load which exceeds your muscle power. Everyone has experienced this sort of painful muscle injury to some extent—as the result of lifting an extremely heavy box, a too strenuous workout in the gym, or from shoveling a ton of snow or dirt.

That said, muscle-strain injuries don't have to occur as a result of a onetime event. They can also occur slowly over time, something medical practitioners refer to as *repetitive strain injuries*. An example of this is when your body's key stabilizing muscles fatigue prematurely during your regular everyday tasks (such as walking or carrying in grocery bags). When a repetitive task proves too much for a "weakling muscle" to handle, another muscle steps in to assist—always to its own detriment—and each time a substitution such as this takes place, you are completely unaware. Until one day, that is—and you get a muscle spasm!

The second scenario for muscle injury occurs when shortened (tight) muscles are forced to lengthen beyond their capacity. As a result their delicate fibers (cells) become frayed. This can happen abruptly—say if you were to fall in an awkward way—or it may come about slowly by way of a different type of repetitive strain injury—one in which your tasks require you to repeatedly extend that shortened muscle to the end of its limited range of motion. A while back I was treating a hardworking mechanic. His lower back muscles were very tight, but his job required him to bend forward countless times throughout his workday. Each time he did—ouch! He pulled on those shortened muscles until they screamed. By following a routine of stretching exercises at home, my patient was able to restore the flexibility to his back muscles, which in turn allowed him to perform his job without wounding his muscles.

Clinical experience has taught me that there are two further problems that come from tight muscles: first, they contribute to bad posture (see chapter 7), and second, over time they tend to result in wear and tear on the joints that live in their neighborhood. Tight and weak muscles *never* make good neighbors.

One of the crucial things to do to restore and maintain our temples is to erect walls against chronic muscle weakness and tightness. The gates to install are the ten exercises that follow. Upon self-evaluation, you may find you need to overhaul some or all of the key muscles I spotlight. Improving your muscle strength and flexibility will prevent you from continually overloading these important muscles just by going about your day. Once normal strength and flexibility have been recaptured, we can place watchmen on our walls by checking from time to time to see if our muscles are still up to par—with a simple run-through of the same exercises.

"Strengthen What Remains…"

Skeletal muscles that have become "downgraded" from lack of use are unable to create the strength of contraction needed to move you or the object you must carry or move. Even the act of standing or sitting up straight requires continuous muscle power. Painful muscle spasms and early fatigue result from weakened muscles that are trying with all their might to do a job beyond their ability. This is not to mention secondary muscle pain, which occurs in the "second-string" muscles that are taking up the slack for the weak "first-string" team. When a muscle is pushed to its limit during physical exertion, it creates a mild to moderately painful sensation (burning, aching, or cramping). This makes it clear to you that it's had enough!

So what exactly must happen to a muscle to make it stronger tomorrow than it is today? While researchers do not have a complete understanding of the entire cause-and-effect process, they do know that muscle cells (fibers) have the ability to divide, as well as to bulk up. In order for muscle growth to happen, a person must challenge their muscle enough (fatigue it with targeted exercise) so a message is sent to the brain reporting that the muscle is not up to the job it needs to perform. Then the brain signals the muscle cells to respond by increasing their size and therefore their power of contraction.[1]

Rules of Engagement: Core Stability

Muscle-strengthening exercises must always be carried out on a stable base, or foundation, in order to avoid injuring other parts of your body. God made provision for that foundation by supplying us with a deep-lying core abdominal muscle called the *transverse abdominus (TA)*. The TA is not one of those "mirror muscles"—you know, the rippling "six-pack" you can see on bodybuilders and other fit athletes. This muscle doesn't even run in the same direction as those others. Its fibers run horizontally, right to left, across your abdomen from the bottom

Transverse abdominus

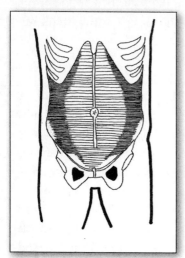

figure 8.3

Multifidus

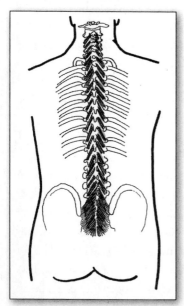

figure 8.4

of your rib cage all the way "south" to where they insert into your pelvic bones (figure 8.3).

When the TA is engaged it causes two other stabilizing muscles to contract along with it—a deep back muscle known as the *multifidus* (figure 8.4) and the group of muscles that make up your *pelvic floor,* or the "bottom" portion of your trunk (figure 8.5). Simultaneous contraction of this muscle trio creates a girdling effect (front, back, and bottom)—a "brace"—which protects against harmful shear forces that would otherwise be transferred to the joints and discs of your spine. Together these three foundational muscles provide better *core protection* as you exercise the other parts of your body.

Case in point: Often when I am reviewing my patients' home exercise program or teaching them a new exercise, they will complain of pain in their back or another nearby joint. By this time they are proficient in performing their abdominal brace, but it has yet to become automatic. When I ask them if they have their "brace" on, they chuckle and admit they forgot. And then they begin again—this time with core stability—and "magically," their associated pain is gone.

Below you will find instructions

on how to retrain your abdominal brace. Dedicate yourself to practicing it so that you will become comfortable and capable of turning your brace "on and off." Then you will be able to use this support system with each of the strengthening exercises that follow (Minutes 1-4).

Pelvic floor

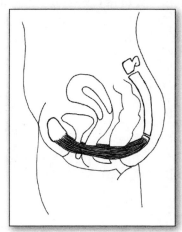

figure 8.5

Transverse Abdominus (TA) Exercise

The first exercise is an abdominal or TA brace. You'll practice it in two positions, the first being in a crawl, on your hands and knees (figures 8.6a and b). If you can't get into this position, it isn't critical. You can begin in the second position (figure 8.7) and still achieve the desired outcome.

Once you're in the crawl position, follow these steps:

1. Relax and allow your abdominal contents to "hang"— see figure 8.6a. (I often place my hand under a patient's stomach and ask them to let me hold their lunch.)

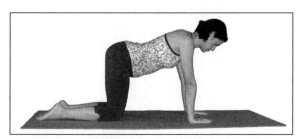

figure 8.6a

2. Take a normal breath *in.*

3. Exhale halfway and pause.

4. Now draw your belly button up toward your spine *without moving your back or your pelvis.* This is the "brace" (figure 8.6b).

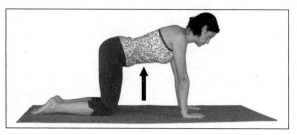

figure 8.6b

5. Exhale fully while maintaining the brace.

6. Continue to breathe normally while maintaining the brace for a cycle of 10 seconds.

7. Repeat steps 1 through 6 ten times (that is, 10 cycles of 10-second bracing while breathing normally).

When you've been able to successfully master an abdominal brace in this crawl position, then try it in the next position, known to physical therapists as hook-lying. Basically, you lie on your back with your knees bent and your feet resting on the floor—see figure 8.7. (This time your hands will be free to monitor your success.)

Beginning in the hook-lying position, follow this sequence of steps:

1. Place your thumbs on the bottom edge of your rib cage, one on each side, as shown in figure 8.7.

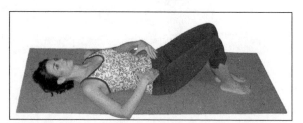

figure 8.7

2. Next place your fingertips in the area of your TA. This can best be felt by first locating the prominent bones you can feel jutting out in the front of your pelvis—your "hip bones." Once your fingertips are on these bony peaks, move them about two inches toward the midline of your body, into the muscle of your abdomen. (If you have some extra padding here, you'll need to push through it.) Your finger tips should now be below the level of your belly button.

3. Before you brace, your TA should feel soft and springy when you push your fingertips into it.

4. With your fingers in place to monitor, take a normal breath *in.*

5. Exhale halfway and pause.

6. Now draw your belly button in toward your spine, away from the front zipper of your pants, *without moving your back or rocking your pelvis.* This, again, is known as the brace.

7. Your thumbs should not feel any rib movement when you "put on" your brace—only after you've begun breathing again.

8. After you brace, your TA should have firmness when you push your fingertips into it—like a tensioned trampoline would feel.

9. Exhale fully while maintaining the brace.

10. Continue to breathe normally while maintaining the brace for a cycle of 10 seconds.

11. Relax, then repeat steps 3 through 7 ten times (that is, 10 cycles of 10-second bracing while breathing normally).

Pelvic Floor Exercise

If you are having difficulty achieving an abdominal brace through the contraction of your TA, you can try to accomplish it by contraction of your pelvic-floor muscles. (Remember, they work together.) If you are a woman and have been pregnant, this will seem familiar to you. Your obstetrician probably taught you Kegel exercises. You were instructed to start and stop your urine flow each time you were urinating. This was to prevent weakening of this muscle group and therefore urine leakage.

While I like the muscular benefit of the "squeeze," I am against messing with the neurological urine-voiding mechanism. Therefore I'd like you to try a *modified* Kegel exercise. Men, you can use the same method and gain the same benefit. Perform the same action you would if you were to shut off your urine stream, only not during actual urination. (If you need to try it a time or two during urination, go ahead. But once you've got the idea, this exercise is best practiced when not in the bathroom.)

Start by attempting the pelvic-floor contraction in the hook-lying position (see figure 8.7). You should be able to feel your TA contract and become firm when you squeeze your pelvic floor. Once you've achieved the abdominal brace (initiated by the pelvic floor), then

1. Continue to breathe normally while maintaining the TA brace for a cycle of 10 seconds.

2. Relax, then repeat ten times (that is, 10 cycles of 10-second bracing while breathing normally).

Whichever way works best for you to initiate the abdominal brace, the goal is for you to be proficient at performing and maintaining it in all positions: hook-lying (lying on your back with your knees bent), side-lying, on hands and knees, sitting, and standing. Ultimately, the goal is for you to be able to use this brace even while walking and performing your daily tasks. Let me assure you that after you've retrained your brace, putting it on will become less and less of a thinking process for you. One day soon it will happen so naturally, you won't even realize you have it on—and that's how God intended it to be!

THE 10-MINUTE MAKEOVER

Minute #1

Target area (muscles): Calves (*gastrocnemius, soleus*)

Exercise: Toe raises

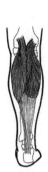

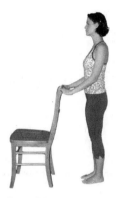
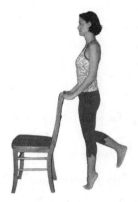

figure 8.8   figure 8.9a   figure 8.9b

Directions:

1. Stand facing a chair back, countertop, or other balancing surface with your feet shoulder-width apart.

2. Place your fingertips on the balancing surface.

3. Brace and breathe.

4. Bend one knee raising your lower leg behind you.

5. Lift your heel off the ground, rising up onto your toes (also commonly known as the "ball of your foot").

6. Slowly lower yourself back down onto your heel, and repeat. (Be mindful not to push yourself up by leaning on your hands and pushing off the balancing surface.)

RIGHT

- Your brace can be maintained throughout the exercise.

- You're rising straight up toward the ceiling as you raise yourself on your toes.

- The exercise results in fatigue sensations in your calf muscle.

WRONG

- You're holding your breath.

- You're leaning forward onto your hands as you raise yourself.

- You're pushing through your hands to bring yourself up.

Goal: 20 reps each leg

Minute #2

Target area (muscles): Lateral hip (*gluteus medius*)

Exercise: Hip drops

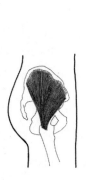

figure 8.10

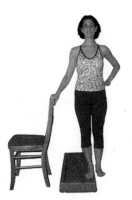

figure 8.11a

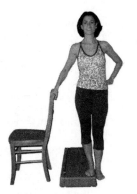

figure 8.11b

Directions:

1. Place a large telephone book (about 2 inches high) or an equivalent on the floor beside something you can hold on to for balance, if you need it at first.

2. Step up onto the book with one foot.

3. Let your other foot make contact with the floor next to the book. (The knee of the "book foot" will be bent at first.)

4. Put on your TA brace and breathe.

5. Straighten the knee of your book foot. This will cause you to lift the heel of your floor foot so only your toes are in contact with the floor.

6. Bend the ankle of your "floor foot" so your toes lose contact with the floor.

7. Place your hand on top of your floor foot hip. Leave your other hand on a balancing surface. (If your balance is good, you can place both hands on your hips.)

8. Now reach your floor foot down toward the floor by letting your hip drop or lower on that unsupported side. Do not allow your "book knee" to bend. Also, maintain the bent-ankle position of the floor foot so the front and back of your foot touch the floor at the same time, not the toes first. When dropping this foot toward the floor you should feel the hand on your hip drop toward the floor as well.

9. When your foot has made light contact with the floor, lift it back up so your hips are once again level.

10. Continue to drop and raise your hip to bring the floor foot into and out of contact with the floor.

11. Stop when fatigued. Switch and perform on the other side.

RIGHT

- Fatigue sensations are felt in the outer hip area of the "book side" only.

- You do not stand or put your body weight on the floor foot—it makes only light contact with the floor. (If you were stepping down onto an ant's back, you would only bend his knees.)

- The "book knee" is bending during the hip-drop phase of the exercise.
- Your hip on the "floor side" is not lowering to the floor along with your foot.

Goal: 15-20 reps each side

Minute #3

Target area (muscles): Buttock (*gluteus maximus*), anterior thigh (*quadriceps*), lateral hip (*gluteus medius*)

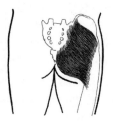
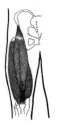
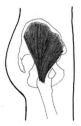

figure 8.12   figure 8.13   figure 8.14

Exercise: Lunges

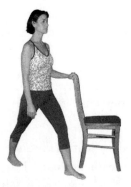
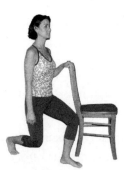

figure 8.15a   figure 8.15b

Directions:

1. Stand beside a countertop or some other surface that can provide hand balance, with your feet shoulder-width apart.

2. Take a large step forward with your left foot.

3. Begin bending your right knee down toward the floor. Your left knee will also bend to "come along for the ride."

4. Slowly lower yourself toward the floor while keeping your trunk upright. (Make sure your left knee does not lean out in front of your left foot. It should be directly over your foot.)

5. When you have lowered yourself as low as you can while still maintaining quality and control of the movement, push through your feet, using your leg muscles to straighten your knees.

6. Repeat until the signs of fatigue set in.

7. Begin again, this time stepping forward with your right foot.

8. Start with a shallow lunge and increase the depth of your lunge as you are able. The lower you drop your back knee, the more difficult the exercise will be to perform.

RIGHT

- Your brace can be maintained throughout the exercise.

- You are able to maintain your balance. Progress to "no hands."

- The exercise results in fatigue sensations in the front of both thighs, usually one more than the other.

WRONG

- You're—guess what?—holding your breath.

- You're wobbling all over the place as you lower yourself.

- You're leaning to the side of your "balance" hand.

Goal: 15-20 reps each leg

(When this goal is achieved, you can challenge yourself further by advancing the depth of your lunge.)

Minute #4—*(Seconds 1 through 30)*

Target area (muscles): Stomach (*rectus abdominus*)

Exercise: Dead bugs

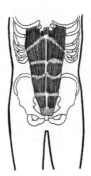

figure 8.16

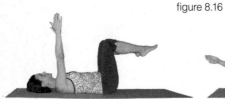

figure 8.17a

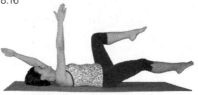

figure 8.17b

Directions:

1. Lie on your back with your arms pointing up to the ceiling.

2. Lift your feet off the floor so your hips are bent at a 90-degree angle.

3. Brace and breathe.

4. Slowly extend your right leg and your left arm out toward the floor—but not all the way.

5. Bring your leg and arm back to the start position, and repeat with your left leg and your right arm.

6. Return to the start position.

7. Once you get used to moving these diagonally opposite limbs together, you can begin to lower one pair while the other pair is still on its way back to the start position. This combined motion gives the "dead bug" its name— you're on your back with all limbs slowly moving at once. (Actually the exercise would be more accurately named the "dying bug.")

*It is extremely important to maintain a stable (nonmoving) spine while you are moving your limbs.

RIGHT

- Your spine is stable, and your brace is maintained.
- Fatigue is felt in your abdomen.
- Your head is resting on the floor.

WRONG

- You're holding your breath.
- Your low back is arching off the floor during limb movements.

Goal: 30 reps, counting each leg "kick out" as "1."

(You can advance this exercise simply by extending your arms and legs farther away from your trunk.)

(Seconds 31 through 60)

Target area (muscles): Chest (*pectoralis major*), arms (*triceps*), and shoulders (*serratus anterior*)

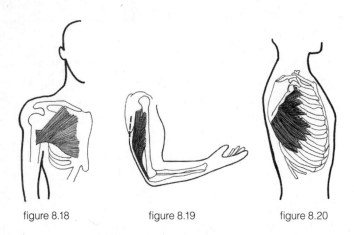

figure 8.18   figure 8.19   figure 8.20

Exercise: Wall push-ups

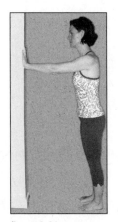   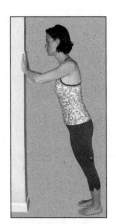

figure 8.21a   figure 8.21b

Directions:

1. Stand facing a wall, with your feet about 1½ to 2 feet from the wall surface.

2. Brace and breathe.

3. Tuck your chin slightly and keep your head ("block 4") drawn back a bit to keep it lined up over your shoulders ("block 3").

4. Lean forward, placing your hands on the wall at the height of your shoulders while keeping your elbows straight.

5. Push your rib cage gently backward until your shoulder blades are snugly seated against your back.

6. Begin bending your elbows, leaning forward toward the wall (just like in a floor push-up).

7. Push through your arms to return to a straight elbow position.

8. You may perform partial elbow bends if you are unable to keep your shoulder blades snug against your back (so they don't lift off your rib cage, or "wing"). Work up to a full range.

RIGHT

- Your brace and your head and neck positions are maintained.
- Your shoulder blades are flush against your back throughout the exercise.
- Fatigue is not typically felt in the shoulder blade area.

WRONG

- Your shoulder blades are "winging."
- You're holding your breath.
- You're leading to the wall with your chin instead of your forehead.

Goal: 15-20 reps. (Challenge yourself by moving your feet farther from the wall, increasing your body's incline.)

Stretch Yourself to New Lengths

Normal life requires a certain amount of muscle flexibility. Without it, everyday living begins to take on a not-so-normal look and feel. As you get older, you'll typically begin to lose some of your God-given stretch-ability. Some of this stiffness is the result of "evaporation." As your body's water content declines as the decades pass, so does the suppleness and extensibility of your muscles. This is because water is one of the key ingredients responsible for the lubrication of the gliding mechanism between muscle fibers which allows for the lengthening of your muscles. (Yet another reason to stay well hydrated.)

Regardless of age, muscles have a tendency to become stiff when you stop fully lengthening them. This condition is known as *adaptive shortening*. To make matters worse, subconsciously your body responds to this limited length by further limiting your movement patterns— the way you bend, or reach for something—so that you are kept within the limitations of your shrunken-down "muscle clothes." Over time this limited movement behavior can lead to the premature breakdown of your muscle and skeletal system, as well as the breakdown of your spinal discs (the "cushions" in between the bones of your spine). So if you want to steer clear of this wear-and-tear zone it is critical that you work to restore and maintain a great deal of the flexibility you had when you were 20 (yes, I did say 20!). You'll be surprised at how quickly the body can remodel itself.

Another significant benefit of good stretch-ability is that it is necessary to regain a healthy, upright posture. Certain muscles must have adequate length in order to regain and maintain the upright postures we talked about in the previous chapter. For instance, tight chest muscles (pectorals) will hold you in a fixed rounded-shoulder physique. And no amount of convincing can win over a tight muscle. They always get their way—that is, until they are stretched!

Adding flexibility to an already damaged body—one with arthritis or something similar—can have very great benefits. One of my former patients is a poster child for the importance of stretching. Roger retired from his law practice with the intention of spending his golden years on the golf course. Unfortunately, his body wasn't playing along.

His back began to ache, and soon, his swing was off. A month later he could no longer walk the course and was having to play only 9 of 18 holes—driving from hole to hole in a golf cart. This was not what he had in mind.

A visit to an orthopedist and a set of X-rays revealed significant arthritis in his low back, with mild to moderate right-hip arthritis as well. His doctor gave him the "you're older now, and must learn to adapt to the aging process" speech. Roger wasn't buying it. He showed up at my office, and within three weeks he was back to his old—but much better—self. And all it took was some focused attention to his muscle flexibility.

Has it been a long time since you've felt limber? Don't waste one more day being an "old stiff"—it's time you restored your temple's mobility. Ready…set…get stretching!

STRETCH-OLOGY: WHAT YOU NEED TO KNOW BEFORE YOU START BENDING

How often should I stretch? The focus of this book is to add quick and easy improvements to your overall health. Therefore in this chapter I am proposing a once a day "10-Minute Muscle Makeover." That said, when I treat patients who are trying to *get out of pain*, I recommend that they *stretch 2 to 3 times per day*.

How much "stretch" should I feel? As you lengthen the muscle, the stretch *intensity* should be about a *5* on a scale of 1 to 10. Not so much that it is painful and not so light that it is comfortable. The muscle needs to feel like it is being stretched. If not, your brain will not get the "lengthen" message. If the stretch intensity is too great, instead of elongating, the muscle under tension will instead contract and try to shorten itself. This is as a means of protection because it believes it may tear under the stress.

What stretching technique should I use? Your stretches need to be performed with a smooth, steady hold. That means *no bouncing*. This is because there are two elements to a muscle: elastic and plastic. Bouncing is absorbed by the muscle's *elastic* element, much like pulling on a rubber band. While the pulling succeeds at stretching the rubber band temporarily, there is no lasting effect on its length.

Muscle length is only truly affected by changing the plastic component of the muscle. Did you ever play with a Slinky as a child? It came tightly coiled in its box from the store. Once you played with it for a while, invariably you would leave it hanging from something for too long. The result was that your Slinky never quite returned to its nicely coiled structure. The Slinky's "plastic element" had been permanently deformed (lengthened). In the body, the plastic element of your muscles is affected only when a lengthened muscle position (a stretch) is held over time, specifically *30 seconds* of time.

What actually occurs when muscles are stretched? Two things happen. Initially, the individual contracting segments (or sarcomeres) that we spoke of earlier are elongated to their full extent. (This is the "elastic" element of the muscle.) Next, the surrounding connective tissue "casings" that encompass the individual muscle cells, cell bundles, and the outside of the muscle itself undergo a reconstructive process. The misaligned collagen fibers that make up much of the casing realign themselves in a more parallel formation, which enhances the stretch-ability of the muscle. This secondary action affects the plastic element of the muscle, giving a more permanent change in length.

Minutes #5-6

Target muscles: Hamstrings

Exercise: Posterior thigh stretch

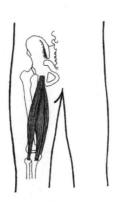

figure 8.22

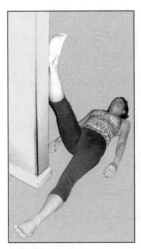

figure 8.23

Benefits package:

- improved forward bending while your knees are straight
- increased step length (on the same side as the stretched muscle)
- decreased shearing force from forced backward bending (extension) in your low back while walking

Directions:

1. Lie on your back with your legs through a doorway (but closer to the right side of the door opening).

2. Lift your right leg and place your right heel immediately to the right of the door opening (usually the molding is there), keeping both your right and left knees straight.

3. Adjust your distance through the doorway (and therefore

how high your heel rests on the wall) based on how strong a stretch you feel in the back of your right thigh (some of you may even feel the stretch down into your calf as well). Too strong? Move further back. Too light? Scoot further through the doorway.

4. Once you have found the correct distance, steadily hold this position.

5. Switch sides and stretch your left leg.

Duration of stretch: Hold for 1 minute, each leg

Minute #7

Target muscles: Iliopsoas, gastrocnemius

Exercise: Anterior hip and calf stretch

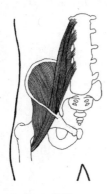
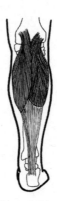
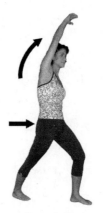

figure 8.24   figure 8.25   figure 8.26

Benefits package:

- Improved ankle and hip range of motion
- Increased step length (on the opposite side)
- Decreased backward bending (extension) force transmission into the lumbar spine while walking

Directions:

1. Take a large step forward with one leg, while making sure both feet remain pointed straight ahead. (Keep both heels on the ground throughout the exercise.)

2. Squeeze your buttock muscles together and "tuck your bottom" (flattening the arch in your lower back).

3. Glide your body forward out over your front foot by bending your front knee. (Make sure not to bend your other knee.) You will begin feeling the stretch in your opposite hip and calf muscles.

4. Reach your arm up over your head (the arm on the same side as the hip and calf muscles you are stretching) and bend your trunk slightly away to increase the stretch in the front of your hip.

   (Need balance? Steady yourself by gently holding onto something with your unraised arm.)

Duration of stretch: Hold for 30 seconds each side

Minute #8

Target muscle: Piriformis

Exercise: Buttock stretch

Benefits package:

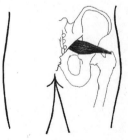

figure 8.27

- elimination of leg pain caused by the sciatic nerve (the nerve that runs down the back of your leg)

- decreased irritation at the muscle-insertion point of the hip (which often leads to hip bursitis pain)

Directions:

1. Lie on your back with your knees bent and your feet on the floor (hook-lying).

2. Cross your right ankle over your left knee (like a man might cross his legs while sitting).

3. Place your right hand behind your right knee and your left hand behind your right ankle. At this point your head should be resting comfortably on the floor. (It has a tendency to lift up so it can peer down at the action.)

4. Simultaneously, lift both your right knee and right ankle up toward your chest while gently directing your right knee across your trunk toward your left shoulder.

5. Stop when you feel a moderate stretch develop in your right buttock, and hold the stretch there.

6. Repeat with left leg.

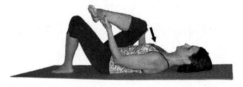

figure 8.28

Duration of stretch: Hold for 30 seconds each side

Minute #9

Target muscle: Upper trapezius

Exercise: Lateral neck stretch

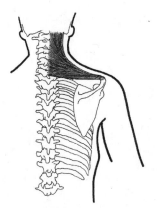

figure 8.29

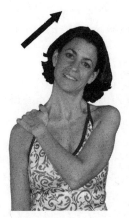

figure 8.30

Benefits package:

- decreased compression on the joints of your neck
- decreased muscle pain that accompanies tightness or spasm
- increased range of motion in your neck; the ability to lower your shoulders to the proper height so you can achieve healthy posture

Directions:

1. In a seated position, reach your left hand across your body and place it on top of your right shoulder.

2. Pull down on your right shoulder, depressing it. (I don't mean making it sad—simply lower it relative to your left shoulder.)

3. While maintaining the downward force on your right

shoulder, slowly side-bend your head to the left, directing your left ear toward your left shoulder.

4. Stop when you feel a stretch in the right side of your neck muscles.

Duration of stretch: Hold for 30 seconds each side

Minute #10

Target muscle: Pectoralis major

Exercise: Chest stretch

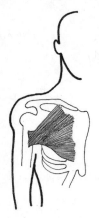 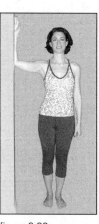 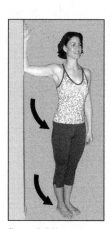

figure 8.31   figure 8.32a   figure 8.32b

Benefits package:

- improved ability to hold your shoulders in the "down and back" position for proper posturing
- decreased pulling on your lower neck (because of slumped posture)
- fewer headaches caused by slumped posture

Directions:

1. Stand next to a doorway or the outside corner of a wall.

2. Place your right forearm on the wall so your elbow is at the same height as your shoulder (see figures 8.32a and b). Your arm should be in line with your body, not in front or behind.

3. Turn your body to the left (away from the wall) by marching your feet in place to face off to the left. Allow the rest of your body to follow your feet. Don't overturn your neck to the left—your nose should stay in line with your breastbone.

4. Stop marching when you feel a stretch in your right front chest area.

5. Repeat on the left.

Duration of stretch: Hold for 30 seconds, each side.

● ● ●

I'm sure you've heard people talk about offering God "the sacrifice of praise." It seems like a virtuous thing to do, but what would constitute it? I believe many things would fit into this category. When you've lost your job and you show up at church to sing praise songs to your Redeemer, if you just received a scary diagnosis from your doctor and you still carry on with your plans to serve on an upcoming missions trip, when your first child goes to college and it squeezes you financially yet you still remain a faithful tither—all these can be opportunities for you to offer God a sacrifice of praise.

Now let me expand that definition somewhat to include something you'd perhaps rather not do, but you submit yourself to it anyway out of obedience to God, because you know it is part of His will for your life. I suggest that physical exercise falls into this category. Physical exercise will cost time, effort, and even mild discomfort. Often you may not even feel like doing it. But the rich reward comes when you do it anyway out of a heart brimming with love and led by obedience. So as you embark on this new and challenging pathway to wellness, keep an attitude of praise in the forefront of your mind so that your sacrifice will be holy and acceptable to the Lord.

NEHEMIAH'S WAY OF PUTTING IT ALL TOGETHER

STEP 1: Cry out to the Lord

STEP 2: Seek His forgiveness

STEP 3: Ask for His empowerment for success

Prayer: *Dear Lord Jesus, I admit that although I knew exercise was good for me, I haven't really been serious about making it a priority in my life. Please forgive me for letting my temple walls fall into disrepair in this regard. I am desperate for You to fill me with the drive and desire to incorporate strength and flexibility training into my weekly routine. I will seek to do this new thing as a sacrifice of praise to You, my King, who have sacrificed everything for me. In the name of Jesus, I pray, Amen.*

STEP 4: Take an honest assessment of your health

1. I presently follow a strength and flexibility program (circle):

   Yes   No

2. I feel weakness or excessive fatigue during the day (circle):

   Never   Occasionally   Sometimes   Frequently   Always

3. The last time I performed strengthening exercises was…
   (circle):

   When I pushed myself out of the womb

   More than five years ago

   Within the last four years

   Just this week

4. I feel stiffness in my body (circle):

   Never   Occasionally   Sometimes   Frequently   Always

5. The last time I performed stretching exercises was…
   (circle):

   > When I reached for my baby bottle

   > More than five years ago

   > Within the last four years

   > Just this week

6. I have pain or disability caused by muscle, disc, or joint
   problems (circle):

   > Yes   No

STEP 5: Verbalize your commitment to change

The person to whom I will verbalize my intent to improve my health
in this area is: _____

STEP 6: Develop a detailed plan of action

I need to perform the following exercises to regain my strength and
flexibility:

1.	6.
2.	7.
3.	8.
4.	9.
5.	10.

STEP 7: Use the buddy system

Someone who would want to join me in making this better-health
change (or who I could trust to keep me accountable) is:

_____

9

Put the Brakes on Brain Aging

The Secret to Keeping Your Mind Sharp, Healthy, and Happy

The end of all things is near. Therefore be clear
minded and self-controlled so that you can pray.

1 PETER 4:7

ack when I was in college, I used to spend Sunday afternoons
visiting with the residents of a local nursing home. I didn't
know much about brain aging back then, but it was certainly
evident from my visits that not everyone's brain aged the same way.
Some of the residents, while reliant on their walkers or wheelchairs to
get around, were mentally sharp and even witty. Others stared straight
ahead, mumbling to themselves and occasionally crying out in a non-
lucid way. The disparity was drastic. Back then, as a biology major who
had studied only genetics up to that point, I assumed that these dif-
ferences had to be due solely to a person's heredity. Shuddering at the
thought that I might end up like some of those who were worse off, I
just hoped that my Creator had dipped into my parents' gene pools
favorably when He designed my brain. (And secretly I hoped that *someone* would still want to spend time with me regardless of how my brain
ended up aging.)

Fast-forward 25 years...my simplistic view of brain aging has been replaced by years of medical research and study. The brain and its workings are a true wonder in every sense. I liken the capacity and complexity to that of the universe. While we can certainly appreciate it for its vastness and complexity, we've only begun to scratch its surface. Scientific exploration and understanding of the brain's mechanisms are still in a stage of relative infancy. Even so, the limited understanding we do have of the brain's structure and function is enough to cause scientists to stand in awe, even if many refuse to accept that a magnificent Creator stands behind it all.

In spite of the vast number of functions of the brain, when we think about aging and its effects on brain health, the areas that come to mind first are *memory, focus,* and *concentration.* And there is good reason for that. Those of us who have entered our forties have likely felt a gradual (albeit subtle) decline in these three areas—enough to begin to worry us just a bit. To mask our concern we laugh about these "senior moments" with friends or family members jokingly dismissing these brain glitches as part of getting old.

But deep inside, "losing our mind" is one of our biggest fears. I know it's one of mine. I watched my own mother succumb to early-onset dementia, which began in her late fifties. *Her* parents also had problems with their minds that became increasingly evident as they aged—my grandmother had Alzheimer's disease for the last dozen years of her life, and my grandfather had dementia that began around his eightieth birthday. Along with the gradual loss of brain function came the eventual loss of their ability to live independently, think rationally, and remain anchored in reality.

I hope to take a new road—one in which my mind remains highly functional all the days of my life. You probably feel the same way, even if you don't have any personal experience with the condition of dementia. Good news—there are some extremely exciting and proven helps for preserving and even regaining lost brain power. In fact, clinical studies have demonstrated these methods of self-treatment to be so effective that Alzheimer's risk can be cut by upwards of 71 percent—reversing the effects of brain aging on cognitive function by a full 7 to 14 years! Now that's something worth working toward, isn't it?

DEMENTIA VS. ALZHEIMER'S DISEASE

Dementia is not a specific disease, but rather a group of symptoms that includes two or more of the following:[1]

- memory loss
- difficulty communicating
- inability to learn or remember new information
- difficulty with planning and organizing
- difficulty with coordination and motor functions
- personality changes
- inability to reason
- inappropriate behavior
- paranoia
- agitation
- hallucinations

Alzheimer's disease (AD), which accounts for 60 to 70 percent of all dementias, can only be diagnosed with 100 percent accuracy post mortem, when the brain itself can be examined for the microscopic *senile plaquing* that characterizes the disease.

Jesus' command to love God with all your mind requires that you have a functioning mind to work with. I am excited to share the specifics I've learned on this topic of brain health so that you too will be empowered to preserve your mind for the tasks you've yet to accomplish for His kingdom's sake. So if you're ready, we'll jump in with both feet—hold onto your skull, because here we go.

What's Inside of My Head?

My daughter asked me the above question at three years of age. Being a science teacher at my core, and thrilled that I had a new student, I went directly to my bookshelf and began thumbing through my old anatomy textbook—the one for the human dissection course I took back in physical therapy school. As I began to show Casey the brain that God had fashioned inside of her skull, I was once again struck with awe as I considered "the works His hands have made." *One hundred billion* brain cells (*neurons*) sit among *one trillion* support cells (*glia*). This vast array of neurons is interconnected throughout the brain by an estimated *one quadrillion* junction points (*synapses*). That's right—the Creator fashioned our brains with an ample 1,000,000,000,000,000 individual connections…can I get a hallelujah, anyone?

Your brain, which makes up only 2 percent of the mass of your body, uses a whopping *20 percent* of its resources. The organ itself has a very soft consistency; slightly firmer than Jell-O—not dense and rubbery as many imagine it to be. It's housed, as you know, in a very hard shell (your skull), which has quite a few sharp bony juts along the inside—something you might not have known. The brain is "aquatic" by nature, as it is continuously bathed in fluid (*cerebrospinal fluid*) both from the inside and the outside. This provides the perfect environment for it to function in.

The exterior of the brain, which is typically known for its folds and convolutions, is called the *cerebral cortex*. Because it is composed of the grayish bodies of the brain's neurons, it is often referred to as the brain's *gray matter* (see figure 9.1 below). The interior portion of the brain is a complex tangle of the tail end, or *axons*, of the brain's nerve cells. Axons are responsible for the relay of messages (in the form of electrical impulses), which run back and forth between the different regions of the brain's gray matter and to the rest of the body as well.

Each messaging axon is wrapped in a whitish insulation called *myelin*. The important role of myelin can be best understood if you know a bit about electrical wiring. At their core, electrical wires contain a metal, such as copper, that easily conducts electrical impulses. But electrical impulses can be "flighty"—jumping off a wire and onto anything that they come in contact with. That is why electrical wires (and the axons in your brain) must be coated with insulation. The insulation keeps the electricity on track and gets it to where it was intended. While electrical wires are coated in colored plastic, your axons are coated in white, waxy myelin. For that reason this interior region of the brain is called the *white matter* (figure 9.1).

Nerve Cell Body (gray matter)

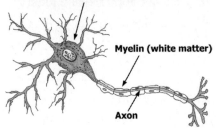

Myelin (white matter)

Axon

figure 9.1

For the purpose of this chapter I want to highlight two specific areas of the brain that are understood to govern the functions which we are striving to preserve—memory, focus, and concentration.

The first portion of your brain to become familiar with is the *frontal cortex* (see figure 9.2), which is located right behind your forehead. It acts as the CEO of your brain and is responsible for executive functions such as decision making, planning, long-term memory, and executing complex actions. (Funny thing— when people are trying to make a thoughtful decision, they often rub their foreheads to "aid" the thinking process.)

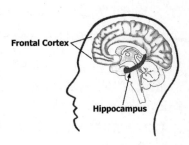

Frontal Cortex

Hippocampus

figure 9.2

The second region of great importance in our discussion of brain aging is an area called the *hippocampus* (see figure 9.2). The hippocampus is actually a paired structure located deep within your brain above and slightly in front of your ears in the region of your "temples." Its claim to fame is that it is the brain's "memory-maker." Every night it judges which of the day's hundreds of events and visual details to place in storage and which to delete. (And again I find it fascinating that when you or I are trying to recall something from the far recesses of our minds, we place our index finger over this area and either rub it or give it a tap or two. It seems we inherently know which part of our brain needs some "massaging.")

Trading In Your Old Brain for a Newer Model

The human brain begins to show signs of deterioration as early as 30 years of age. This process is marked by a progressive breakdown of neuron connections within the gray matter. By the time you reach your forties, your brain cell loss begins to pick up some serious speed. That's where I am, and I most certainly feel the effect my age has had on my brain cells. Here's a list of my own "mental deficiencies":

- walk into a room and forget why I came
- cannot recall a conversation I've had with an immediate family member (which likely occurred while I was thinking about something else)
- lose my train of thought…sometimes mid-sentence
- can't locate the exact word I'm looking for in order to accurately express myself

Sound familiar, anyone? When I was a teenager there was a TV commercial that showed a close-up of an egg being fried in a hot skillet. The caption read, "This is your brain on drugs." It used to pop into my mind often when my kids were young—although I had personalized it to read, "This is your brain on toddlers"…but I digress. Today, if you're like me, you may struggle with the fact that your brain feels "fried" after a grueling day at work, when trying to juggle too many tasks, or even when just trying to have a conversation with a friend!

Praise God, I am happy to report that human brain cells can be *regained, retrained,* and *maintained.* And just like in other areas of health, much of the future integrity of our minds depends on the choices we make each day. Would it surprise you to find out that there might be things you neglect to do, thoughts you think, and foods that you may be eating that actually speed up that aging process? Throughout this chapter I'll point out these hazardous things so you can know where to erect walls to keep these harms out of sight and out of your mind.

Scientific studies have now given us concrete direction by identifying particular foods and activities that act to *protect* the integrity of the brain's neurons, and therefore prevent or slow the brain's decline as we age. By utilizing these brain-support tactics, we can bolster our brain power by creating a "brain reserve." Much like the U.S. Army Reserve, a brain reserve provides back up forces (extra brain cells) that can move into frontline position if and when needed.

According to Paul E. Bendheim, MD, the author of *The Brain Training Revolution*, brain reserves provide us with alternate thought "routes" in the event that the "main road" is out of service. By equipping ourselves with the knowledge of how to protect our brain cells, and by installing appropriate gates to allow healthful practices into our lives, we can effectively prolong the sharpness of our minds and help prevent the occurrence of Alzheimer's disease and other dementias.

Sharpen Your Mind While You Sleep

Anyone who has suffered though a restless night has felt the immediate impact of that one sleepless night on their mental capacity. Thoughts are slowed along with reaction time, and any thinking that requires some higher level of focus or computation is a real struggle. Not to mention that your mood throughout the day is somewhat depressed, isn't it? Back in chapter 4 we talked about the five stages of sleep that occur within each 90-minute sleep cycle, and how specific actions take place in the body during each of those phases. Without a full 7 to 8 hours, less time is spent in stages 3 through 5, which is harmful to your brain on many levels (You will probably recall several of these issues from chapter 4).

The first problem with being "underslept" is that it is during the non-REM and REM sleep stages that the brain's neurotransmitters and hormones such as serotonin, dopamine, endorphins, and norepinephrine are replenished. Without sufficient quantities of these critical substances, your brain will not function as your Designer intended. Moods, energy levels, even body weight are negatively influenced.

Habitually getting less than seven hours of sleep a night produces harmful effects on numerous other processes that are critical for optimal brain health. It has been discovered that sleep-deprived people actually have lower activity in the temporal lobes of their brains—the home of the hippocampus (your memory maker).[2] So less sleep equals poorer memory. Sleep deprivation also affects the frontal cortex (your decision maker and high-level thinker).[3] As a result thinking becomes dulled and inefficient. Still another study found that people were less effective at making executive decisions after missing just *one night* of sleep.[4] If you struggle with indecision or making poor decisions, according to this study, sleep can make you wiser!

Another activity that happens while you're sleeping is the process of *neurogenesis*, or new brain cell (neuron) production. It is critical to your brain health—both for the day and long-term—that none of this neuron manufacturing time is lost. Without adequate creation of new brain cells, you can't keep up with the brain cell loss you suffer each day. Neurogenesis is stimulated by a substance called *brain-derived neurotrophic factor*, or BDNF. Multiple research studies have shown that sleep deprivation lowers BDNF levels, in essence creating a "work slowdown" in your brain's factory, which ultimately limits your body's ability to maintain your mental capacity.

Sleep also offers your brain *"rehearsal time"* to review newly performed tasks. When you learn a new computer program at work, your brain will practice the new procedures over and over again while you sleep. The next day, you will have the added benefit of having reviewed all night long. In addition, your brain performs the task of *memory consolidation* while you slumber. This takes place in the hippocampus which sorts through the day like yesterday's mail, deciding which memory to throw away and which to keep.

Have you ever used the expression "Let me sleep on it" when trying to come to a decision about something? No wonder! While you are soundly snoozing, your brain uses this precious time to *analyze*, *problem-solve*, and even *learn*.[5] Maybe you've experienced this yourself when you've gone to bed with a problem you couldn't solve, and awakened "magically" with the answer. For myself, I always found that in college if I studied well but got to bed before midnight I performed much better than if I had stayed up all night to cram for my exam. I guess my brain was busy reviewing while I was getting some shut-eye.

Here's what you can take away from this section: You can grab hold of this sleep-induced brain aid by just getting to bed earlier. And, honestly, who doesn't like to sleep? It's effortless, it's free, and it's readily available. Choose to install the sleep gate for better brain health and a brighter tomorrow.

ARE YOU BREATHING WHILE YOU'RE SLEEPING?

The condition known as *sleep apnea* has been increasingly covered in the media. People with sleep apnea literally stop breathing for brief periods—multiple times throughout the night (sometimes upwards of 30 times an hour). This disorder places them at high risk for many diseases such as heart and brain attacks (stroke), high blood pressure, obesity, and type 2 diabetes.

So how does sleep apnea affect your mental capacity? The problem with not breathing as much as you should throughout the night is that your brain becomes oxygen-starved. Without adequate oxygen, your brain cells will die off at a much faster rate. Elevated blood pressure (which often accompanies sleep apnea) can also lead to microscopic strokes that kill off small portions of your brain matter. Sleep apnea is also associated with depression, which will leave both your brain and your life in a fog.

If you are significantly overweight, wake up excessively tired each day, or if your spouse tells you that you snore loudly, stop breathing, or make choking or gasping sounds throughout the night, *please* get yourself to a sleep center. There is an easy fix to this problem, and you will look, feel, and think so much better...and you'll live longer too.

Feed Your Head

In terms of food, a heart-healthy diet is a brain-healthy diet. Free radicals pose a large problem within your head, as they do throughout your entire body. These "radicals" try to overthrow and undermine your brain function and integrity. Therefore, eating foods rich in antioxidants (berries, citrus, almonds, broccoli, and so on) is a must if you are to combat the aging affects of free radicals. A large study out of Chicago's Rush Institute for Healthy Aging found that those who eat *three servings* of vegetables each day slowed their intellectual decline by 40 percent when compared to those who those who avoided veggies.[6] A fabulous study published in 2006 from Columbia University found that people who adhered to a "Mediterranean Diet" (one rich in vegetables, nuts, olive oil, etc,) cut their risk of Alzheimer's by an amazing *68 percent.*[7]

A brain healthy diet must also include *omega-3 fatty acids.* If you recall from the beginning of this chapter, each "tail part," or axon, of your brain's cells is coated in a white, waxy material called myelin. This insulation material suffers wear and tear from transmitting electrical messages to and from your brain all day long. Myelin is made from fatty acids and can be easily replenished by eating omega-3 powerhouse foods, such as salmon, walnuts, and olive oil (see chapter 5 to refresh your memory on antioxidants and omega-3 fatty acids).

Fatty acids also comprise much of your brain cells' membranes— the skin that holds the entire neuron together. In 2006, Tufts University published a study that showed that adults who eat seafood three times per week (especially varieties known to be high in omega-3's) deceased their risk of Alzheimer's disease by 39 percent.[8] So pick up a fishing pole or stop by your local fish market for a real brain boost!

WATER YOUR BRAIN

Water is essential for brain health because your brain is basically a lightweight sponge made up of 80 percent water. Not only that, but it sits bathed in cerebrospinal fluid, 90 percent of which is H_2O. So drink up— and if you find water to be a "boring" beverage—add some interest with a slice of citrus fruit, or heat it up and turn it into tea. (Did someone say tea? I'll be right over!)

Optimal brain health requires attention not only to what you eat but to *how much* you eat as well. In other words, you must trim down to smarten up. According to Dr. Daniel Amen, the author of *Making A Good Brain Great*, the risk of getting dementia is *three-and-a-half times greater* for people whose BMI (body mass index) is either overweight or obese than for those who fall into the normal BMI range.[9] (If you're wondering what your BMI is and you haven't read chapter 6, visit my website, www.LisaMorrone.com, to use a free BMI calculator.)

However, if you follow the dietary suggestions from chapters 5 and 6 and install gates for premium fueling and erect walls against empty or excessive calories, then you will find you have all the nutritional resources in place to regain, retrain, and maintain your precious brain cells.

Take Your Brain Out for a Walk

I have to say it again—wellness *requires* exercise. Study after study confirms that what is good for your skeletal muscles is good for your "mental muscle." Women who perform moderate exercise just 90 minutes per week show a 20 percent decreased risk in memory and attention span loss.[10] For people who spend regular time exercising, a U.S. study showed participants to have a *38 percent* less chance of developing dementia and an Italian study showed *71 percent* less chance.[11] (Maybe those fabulous European results had to do with the Mediterranean diet—see chapter 5.)

Another study showed it is never too late to gain brain benefit from exercise. A group of newly-exercising 71-year-old men who were studied over a six-year period were found to have a *50 percent* decrease in dementia occurrence.[12] I don't know about you, but I've found a new motivation to keep moving for as long as my good Lord will enable me! (If back or neck pain are limiting factors in your ability to get up and go, pick up a copy of my book *Overcoming Back and Neck Pain* and gain control over your pain by learning to treat it yourself.)

But why does physical exertion have this positive effect on the brain? There are a number of reasons.

- First, exercise *improves blood flow* throughout the body. Since the brain uses 20 percent of the body's resources, the better your overall circulation, the more nourishment and oxygen the brain can get hold of.
- The second effect exercise has on the brain comes from the somewhat stressful, taxing affect that

moderate-to-high-level exercise has on the body. This physical stress actually prompts *an increase in the production of BDNF*—the brain's version of Miracle-Gro.

- In addition, exercise seems to kick the brain into spring-cleaning mode. Your brain cells' support team (the glial cells) *tidy up waste products* left behind by everyday brain cell wear-and-tear, leaving fewer free radicals and other pollutants hanging around to fog up your thought processes.

- Exercise has also been found to *ramp up the production of endorphins, serotonin, dopamine, and other good-for-your-brain hormones and neurotransmitters.*

- Lastly, regular exercise adds the benefits of *lower blood pressure, lower body weight, and improved blood sugar metabolism*—all good news for your brain, which works best in a regulated, healthy environment.

You can supercharge the effect of exercise on your brain by "mixing it up" a bit. The brain loves to figure things out (which is how you fortify your mental muscle). So learn to dance, take up tennis, whatever you choose…alternate between different forms of activities. The more complex the movements, the more your brain expands its reserves.

AVOIDING BRAIN DAMAGE

Your soft brain is no match for your hard skull—especially those internal bony peaks that jut out sharply in its direction. Each time you strike your head, your brain gets two injuries: one at the point of contact, and one on the opposite side where it rebounds back against your skull. Recent studies have revealed the massive brain damage football players and boxers have incurred as a result of participating in their sports. Even more disturbing is their increased risk of dementia and Parkinson's disease.

Protect your brain as if your life depended on it, because it does. Always wear a helmet while bicycling, rollerblading, skating—or wherever you are at increased risk of falling. Wear your seat belt at all times in a car (because your brain is no match for your dashboard or windshield). Lastly, steer yourself and your kids clear of sporting activities where repetitive head trauma is expected (for example, heading the ball in soccer, using your head to stop your opponent in football, or using your head as an allowable target in boxing). You will only own one brain in this life; handle it with care!

Mental Gymnastics

Remember when your kindergarten or grade-school teacher used to say, "All right, class, I want everyone to put on their thinking caps"? That used to really bug me. You see, I took it as an insult, as if we were all just sitting around on our mats, dull as our pencils, waiting for snack time. (I know—I was a cynical five-year-old.) Well, if my teacher were still alive today, I'd have to call her up and apologize for my bad attitude. What Mrs. Hall was preparing us to do was *deliberately* challenge our brains' capacity. I should have been grateful.

The effect that intentional higher learning and mental manipulation have on the brain is critical for amassing ample brain reserve. Personally, I have never enjoyed crossword or Sudoku puzzles (probably because I can never finish them), and I don't play mind-teasing video games of any sort. When it comes to math computations, I usually reach for my calculator—even when I can do the math in my head. I don't even challenge myself to learn phone numbers anymore. I just plug 'em into my cell phone. (I don't even know my own kids' numbers by heart—I know that's pathetic, but I'm just being real here.) I've let myself become a "lamebrain" in many ways. Maybe you're starting to feel the same conviction I am. Like I've said before, health is a journey, not a destination. So if your brain has been in neutral, take up the challenge with me, and let's seek to expand our minds.

Mental exercise builds brainpower by manufacturing new connections between neurons (synapses) and strengthening existing ones, and by bulking up cognitive reserves. It enables us to think faster, learn more, and forget less. In order to be effective, mental exercise must challenge your memory, focus, and concentration. A study sponsored by the National Institute of Aging at the National Institutes of Health resulted in an amazing finding: 70-year-olds who were put through a ten-session cognitive training program remembered things more clearly, processed information more speedily, and reasoned more efficiently, to the equivalent of *knocking 7 to 14 years* off their brain age. And the full effect of those ten sessions was still present *a full two years later!* Even five years after that they still maintained their mental advantage.[13]

There are many ways brain training can be implemented. *Reading and writing* are easy ways to add to your brain reserves. (This means more than romance novels and food lists.) *Puzzling, analyzing, and problem-solving* are all potent vitamins for your brain matter. Play the game Concentration with your children or grandchildren, work on the crossword puzzle in your daily paper, visit your local bookstore and pick up one of the many brainpower books and workbooks available. Put down the calculator and use the fleshy one inside your head. And another thing—make it a goal to memorize your children's cell phone numbers (note to self)!

Emotions That Chow Down on Your Gray Matter

Stress, anxiety, and depression—a dreadful threesome. Sometimes they arrive together, sometimes one at a time. We've all experienced at least the first two. And one in six adults in the United States suffers from depression at one time or another during their lifetime. As awful as these problems are to deal with on an emotional level, their affects don't end there. They are actually harmful to your gray matter.

When we talked earlier about the stress of exercising having a positive influence on your brain, that kind of stress is moderate in degree and short-lived. *Chronic life stress* is a whole other story. Brain scans have found that not only does prolonged stress damage brain cells in the hippocampus (your "learner" and "memory maker"), but it also decreases production of BDNF (your brain cell "fertilizer") and increases the production of norepinephrine and dopamine, which cause the misfiring of neurons when the brain is attempting to store long-term memories and direct complex tasks.[14]

Anxiety and depression affect the brain in much the same way. Likely that is why there is a *twofold increase* in the risk of dementia for those who have suffered from clinical depression at some point in their life.[15]

What do you do if your life has more than its fair share of stress? Get help. Seek counsel, learn relaxation techniques, pray, pray, pray… God knows what it is like to be us—frail, sometimes frightened human beings. And He is fully capable of carrying the loads of stress that life often dumps on our doorsteps. And oh, my dear friend—He is ever so faithful!

CHEER UP YOUR BRAIN WITH SOME TLC

Recently I took a continuing education course on the subject of depression. I was pleasantly surprised to learn that two extremely important neurotransmitters, which are found to be at insufficient levels in people suffering with depression, could be produced during particular social settings.

A research study showed that when one person does an act of kindness toward another, both the helper and the one who is helped gained increased levels of both serotonin and endorphins. Even more surprising was that if a third person—an uninvolved bystander—witnessed this act of kindness, *his* levels of serotonin and endorphins increased as well! I guess I shouldn't be that surprised, because Proverbs 11:25 tells us, "A generous man will prosper; he who refreshes others will himself be refreshed." So refresh your brain today…show someone a little TLC!

As that old TV commercial used to remind us, *A mind is a terrible thing to waste.* Let's not lose time installing the brain-healthy gates of adequate sleep, good nutrition, physical exercise, mental calisthenics, and stress management…and remember to wear your helmet!

STEP 1: Cry out to the Lord

STEP 2: Seek His forgiveness

STEP 3: Ask for His empowerment for success

Prayer: *Dear Lord Jesus, I am amazed at everything that goes on in this head of mine. Lord, I don't want to lose my mental capacity as I age. I ask Your forgiveness for the things I have done or not done (knowingly or unknowingly) that have worked against retaining my brainpower. Today I ask that You would give me determination to implement this new information I've just learned—to do the things that will preserve my mind so I can remain a sharp tool in Your hand, my Master. In the name of Jesus, I pray, Amen.*

STEP 4: Take an honest assessment of your health

1. On average I get _____ hours of sleep a night.

2. My dietary intake of antioxidant and omega-3-rich foods (circle):

   Needs major improvement

   Could use some tweaking

   Is pretty good

3. I exercise (circle):

   What's that?

   Once/week

   Twice/week

   3-5 times/week

   6-7 times/week

4. I engage in mentally challenging activities (circle):

Never Occasionally Sometimes Frequently Consistently

5. I suffer from stress, anxiety, or depression (circle):

Never Occasionally Sometimes Frequently Consistently

6. I protect my head from unexpected or unnecessary trauma (circle):

Never Occasionally Sometimes Frequently Consistently

STEP 5: Verbalize your commitment to change

The person to whom I will verbalize my intent to improve my health in this area is: _____

STEP 6: Develop a detailed plan of action

I plan to make the following changes in my life to regain, retrain, and maintain my brain cells:

1.

2.

3.

4.

5.

STEP 7: Use the buddy system

Someone who would want to join me in making this better-health change (or who I could trust to keep me accountable) is:

_____

PART 3

BUILT TO LAST

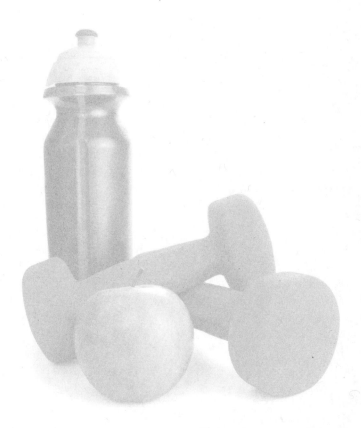

Retirement—Moses' Style
Live Long and Serve Strong

Even in their old age they will still produce
fruit; they will remain vital and green.

PSALM 92:14 NLT

Whenever someone mentions the word *retirement*, images of golf, warm-weather senior communities, and comfort shoes flood my mind. I guess it's because I grew up in a society that has trained me to think of senior citizens as leisure-time beings, past their productive prime—just kicking back, finally getting to enjoy the fruits of their labor. Maybe you've been similarly influenced to see retirement in this way (sort of like a receiving a reward at the end of a job well done).

Over the past decade, however, I've come to realize that our culture has been conditioning its citizens to take part in a very nontraditional, nonbiblical view of retirement. Instead of encouraging older folks to mature into the roles of mentor, teacher, or elder, society has convinced people that when they grow older it would be in everyone's best interest if they would kindly move aside and let the younger generation handle things. While we're encouraged to remain productive throughout the middle portion of our lives, we're also taught to look forward to the time when we can rightfully "quit"…sometime around the age of 65.

Today retirement has become the sought-after prize, the goal, or the victory lap of working people in industrialized nations. But have we all been duped? The very definition of the word *retire* describes a situation that is anything but desirable. It literally means "to withdraw, to fall back or retreat, to remove from active service…usually because of age." That sounds pretty depressing, doesn't it? And yet somehow you and I have been convinced to pine for this stage of life.

So what should our response as Christ-followers be, knowing that we are often called to live in contrast to the world? Is there a sound basis for living outside the lines, or challenging the status quo when it comes to retiring? As with all other aspects of our lives, we need to investigate the word of God to understand the mind of God.

In the Beginning…

…there was no retirement. Men and women worked all their lives until their bodies could no longer go on. Only then did they sit back and let others do for them. Still, just because they lacked the physical strength to be productive, that didn't mean it was time to retire from their role as mentor or wise sage. Jacob, who was blind toward the end of his lifetime, was still giving out verbal blessings, and King David, who was ultimately confined to his bed and given the human version of a heating blanket, continued to prayerfully intercede for his nation. So it shouldn't come as a surprise that God doesn't have a retirement age in mind for you either. Certainly He realizes that you and I may slow down as we age (thanks to the decay of a fallen creation). Even still, the thought of humans "retiring" from kingdom work never crossed the Lord's mind. He sees your life as a continuum of service motivated by your love for Him. In fact, he has been carefully grooming you for the tasks you've yet to accomplish—*all for heaven's sake.*

While it's true that disease and deterioration may require *some* people to be pulled out of circulation, we cannot sit idly by and allow our bodies to race toward decay—especially when so much of how you and I turn out in the end depends upon how we live our lives today and tomorrow. May we have the same mind-set that David did when he proclaimed this to the Lord:

> Since my youth, O God, you have taught me,
> and to this day I declare your marvelous deeds.

> Even when I am old and gray, do not forsake me,
> O God, till I declare your power to the next
> generation, your might to all who are to come.
>
> PSALM 71:17-18

David got it. His job was not complete the day his hair became gray. As long as he had strength in his body and soundness of mind he knew he was charged with the task of declaring God's power to those who came after him.

Each of us has a unique life-message that can powerfully declare to the next generation that God is almighty, all-sufficient, and ever-present. He always keeps His promises—we've lived long enough to experience that. Brothers and sisters, we must make sure we are capable of relaying all we've seen and learned to those who come after us. This is how it is shown throughout the Bible. Stories and life lessons were taught by the elder to the younger. So if the idea of retirement was not God's idea or intention, where did this modern concept come from?

Man's Bright Idea

Retirement had its humble beginnings in Germany. In 1883, Chancellor Otto von Bismarck came up with the idea of *paying* seniors to get them to step out of the workforce. The age he set for this reimbursed retirement? Sixty-five. However, at that time in history, very few individuals actually survived long enough to receive this "benefit."

But as medical treatment advanced, people began living longer past their physical prime. This began to have a negative effect on businesses. Older folks were still occupying jobs that could be filled by younger, cheaper, more "productive" workers. To combat this problem, in 1935, a politician from the sunny state of California initiated a popular movement proposing mandatory retirement for all workers at the age of 60. In exchange, the state's government would pay pensions of up to $200 a month (an amount equivalent at the time to a full salary for a middle-income worker). Dismayed at the prospect of California's radical generosity toward seniors, President Franklin D. Roosevelt proposed the Social Security Act of 1935, which made workers pay for their own old-age insurance.[1]

These days retirement from the workplace is accepted by most people as the way life is supposed to "wind down." We have retirement packages, retirement plans, retirement homes, retirement benefits… all so that we can move out of the way and let someone younger take our place. It may be arguable that in the workforce this practice could be beneficial, but it most certainly does not have the same effect when applied to the kingdom of God. Without the contributions of the aged, the spiritual warfare we are engaged in here on earth suffers. King Solomon attested to this when he pointed out,

> The gray hair of experience is the splendor of the old.
>
> PROVERBS 20:29 NLT

Yet today, many of us cover up our gray, having been conditioned to be ashamed of the signs of aging. (I'm guilty of this.)

Most aging believers today have allowed the concept of retirement from *paid* employment to seep into other areas of their lives—including their God-ordained service to the church and to the world. For many years I ran the vacation Bible school program at my church. Many times I've had senior church members tell me how they used to serve in this or that, but now that they are "retired," they've stepped back to "give someone else a chance." My internal response is, *Are there so few positions for service available today that people have to vacate them in order for others to have a turn?* There's no doubt that the younger members of the church have the energy to work hard, but it's our elders who have the wisdom to work *smart*. Put those two traits together and you have a powerful force! We need everybody on this team—especially those 65 and older. We need their wisdom, their perspective, their patience, their guidance, their experience…in a word, we need them to stay in the game.

God's Plan for Your Sunset Years

Think of our lives as being played out in trimesters. The first 25 to 30 years are the *gathering stage*. We gather the tools we need to use throughout our lives, such as education, interpersonal skills, and job experience.

Our enthusiasm is often matched by unlimited energy resources. (It's no wonder most of the major revolutionaries in history began their "uprisings" during this time in their lives.) If you gave your life to Jesus in this first trimester, you are working out the various aspects of your faith for the first time—learning what it means to make God the center of your life. Let's liken it to the soil preparation time in farming.

The second trimester is the *implementing stage*. Between the ages of 25 or 30 and about 50 or 60 we use all that we've "gathered" during our first trimester and attempt to apply it in building our families, our faith, our careers, and our service avenues. For seasoned believers, it's during this stage we begin to discover exactly what ministry roles God has crafted us to fill, after having served in many "worker bee" roles through the years. With each passing decade the "implementer" who is striving to serve the Lord with his or her life feels more comfortable with the person he or she has been created to be and with the plan God is working in and around them. It's during this stage of life that "crops" have been planted and are seen springing up from the ground and maturing to the point of bearing fruit.

The final trimester of our lives is the *reaping stage*. And while it doesn't really have an exact end point, we can say it spans the time between the age of 50 or 60 up through age 75 to 90. (Although by following the healthy lifestyle suggestions in this book, who knows how long you could live to serve the King?) It is during this final third of life when the fruit of our labors is ripe for the picking. In other words, we glean the reward from our earlier investments. The harvest that results during this time period enables us to share abundantly with others. This bounty includes time, talents, resources, and wisdom—the kind that mentors, leads, and offers instruction to the next generation.

My favorite time of the day is sunset—that is when the sky is filled with glorious and inspirational hues and patterns. Sometimes at the end of the day, clouds blanket the sky and do not allow us to look to the heavens. Let's make sure we work toward using this last stage in our lives wisely—rather than expiring behind a cloud of illness we've cloaked ourselves in, may we leave this world with a great display, pointing others to the magnificence of the Savior.

Remember, retirement is man's design, not God's. Scripture is always faithful to show us the intentions of our Creator. It has provided us with real-life examples of people who, during this "reaping stage" of their lives, embodied Jesus' design and purpose for their old age. By considering three of these God-fearing, God-honoring lives we will gain a clearer picture of what the Savior intends for ours. Following each biblical example, I will introduce you to a twenty-first-century person who is living out their life the way God intended. Although their roles are different, take note of their unique callings, their physical and mental strength, and their obedience to the direction of the Holy Spirit. I hope you come away as inspired as I was when I finished interviewing these amazing saints.

Moses of Old

Most of Moses' "gathering" years were spent in Egypt, where he was raised by Pharaoh's daughter after she had rescued him from the river. Taught by the finest instructors, Moses grew in knowledge and wisdom. Soon after he realized he was an Israelite, his life of grandeur ended, and he entered his implementing stage—out in the fields tending sheep for his father-in-law in the land of Midian. (I guess you could say this was Moses' "Midian-life crisis.") There he spent the next 40 years until one day, through a burning bush, God called Moses to serve him. He was 80 years old.

How many of us even recognize this as a possibility now—a brand-new life calling at 80? Moses entered this last trimester of his life by faithfully serving his Lord, leading his people out of Egypt, instructing them in God's commandments, and bringing them to the threshold of the Promised Land. When God called Moses home at the end of his life, Deuteronomy 34:7 had this to say:

> Moses was a hundred and twenty when he died,
> yet his eyes were not weak nor his strength gone.

Now that's some epitaph!

A Modern-Day Moses

David Bingham recently celebrated his eighty-second birthday.

Raised in a devout Christian home in the Northeast, Dave grew up attending Sunday school and church. Following his mother's advice, he entered Bible college after completing high school. Graduation, however, did not lead him into a pulpit. Rather, Dave sadly recounts, he walked away from his calling and instead spent years "sowing his oats" in the military and the civilian world. After marrying at the age of 27, Dave was ready to return to his spiritual roots. Along with his wife and three children, he faithfully attended church where he taught Sunday school to junior-high boys for over 35 years. Throughout his life he has also served as a church elder, Boys' Brigade leader, and children's church facilitator.

Outside of Sundays, Dave admits to having worked for "fifty years, day and night, six days a week" up until the time he sold his company, just four years ago. His business success has enabled him to live comfortably, but more importantly, he says, to fund the work of God on this earth in significant ways. As part of his stock portfolio, Dave has a "Benevolent Fund" that is specifically earmarked for offerings (beyond his tithe).

Mr. Bingham embodies many of the teachings of this book. He has been a lifelong athlete and has remained trim throughout his adulthood, and even though he had to replace his daily six-and-a-half-mile runs with hour-and-a-half walks two years ago, Dave has continued to keep his temple physically prepared to do the work of the Lord. These days Dave combines exercise with evangelistic outreach down at the local boardwalk. His bright smile and sparkling blue eyes draw people to him, and he freely shares the good news with all who will listen. In addition to physical exercise, Dave works out his mind every day, studying God's Word, memorizing Scripture, and doing crossword, word scramble, and Sudoku puzzles.

Dave has successfully broken his family's pattern…which seemed to take the lives of the men at the age of 65. Good for him! And good for you and me that we have such an encouraging example of the benefits of staying on this journey of health throughout our lifetimes. Dave's life verse is Proverbs 3:5-6: "Trust in the Lord with all thine heart; and lean not unto thine own understanding. In all thy ways acknowledge him, and he shall direct thy paths" (KJV). Amen!

MEET MAYOR McCALLION

Up north in Ontario, a little southwest of Toronto, lies Canada's sixth-largest city, Mississauga. It is governed by a mayor who has been in office some 35 years. More amazing is that Mayor Hazel McCallion first took office at the age of 53! Today Hazel is a vibrant, active 88-year-old woman who is so popular with her constituents that at the last election she swept up 92 percent of the vote.

Each day Hazel remains active, working out in the gym, duck bowling, or donning a pair of ice hockey skates and "dropping a few pucks" (accurately) into the goal. (She was a professional ice hockey player in her twenties—nearly six decades ago!) There seems to be a timeless fount of energy in this remarkable woman.

When asked why she doesn't retire, Mayor McCallion said, "What would I do?" and then without pause, she launched off to explain the important challenges she was currently working on to improve her city's future. If you think this mayor is just leaning back at her desk sipping Ensure, think again. Hazel has managed her city so well that it runs debt-free—with $70 million in reserves. What a great example of blessing the next generation...*You go, girl!*

Caleb of Old

Following in the footsteps of Moses was a man from the very next generation of Israelites, Caleb. When Caleb was 40 years old (early in the implementing stage of his life), Moses asked him to join Joshua and eight other men on a mission to secretly scout out the Promised Land. Caleb and Joshua returned with glowing reports of the land and a fervent zeal for Israel to advance immediately and take the land God had promised to give to them.

However, the other eight spies saw things differently. They had promptly lost their courage after viewing the dauntingly fortified cities and seeing the size of the people who inhabited the land—who they reported to be "giants." This anxious group convinced the people to rebel against Moses and Aaron and refuse to enter the Promised Land—diverting the nation of Israel, yet again, from the will of God.

Because Caleb believed God would be true to His Word, and because he tried to encourage his countrymen to walk by faith and not by sight, God singled out both him and Joshua as the only people of their generation who would live to inhabit the Promised Land. After Moses' death, the Bible tells us that Joshua became the new leader of Israel. Caleb, his right-hand man, was 85 years old when he asked Joshua for his promised "land grant" in Canaan—the city of Hebron. Here is where we read Caleb's account of his own physical condition:

> Here I am today, eighty-five years old.
> I am still as strong today as the day Moses sent me out;
> I'm just as vigorous to go out to battle now as I was then.
>
> Joshua 14:10-11

Wow—to be a "buff" 85-year-old, ready to serve his country in battle! Today, friends, our battlegrounds have changed. We believers are fighting for the souls of the next generation. It has been said that Christianity is only one generation from extinction. Let's do all we can to make sure we are well enough to engage in this battle at 85 and beyond!

A Modern-Day Caleb

Albert Thuro has overcome many obstacles in his life to become the servant of God he is today. Born in Yugoslavia (present-day Serbia) back in 1934, Albert spent seven of his formative years in a refugee camp in Germany, where food was scarce and education was nonexistent. When he was 14 years old, with only six years of formal education under his belt, he began a four-year apprenticeship with a master toolmaker in Germany.

By the age of 21, Albert had mastered his craft so well and showed such promise that he was put in charge of running a tool factory in what was then East Germany, then under Socialist/Communist rule. Aware that socialism never bred wealth, Albert came to the United States in 1956—unable to speak, read, or write a word in English. Here

Mr. Thuro served in the U.S. Army for two-and-a-half years, got married, and began a family and a business—a machine tooling factory. No surprise there.

Nutrition, exercise, and the pursuit of a healthy lifestyle was not part of Albert's first trimester of life—survival was all that mattered. However when he married at the age of 25 and his wife became his "meal provider," he did note that she cooked well-balanced meals with plenty of vegetables, and that she would portion out the food on everyone's plate and then serve her family their pre-portioned plates at the dinner table. There were no second helpings or bottomless bowls of food brought to the table—a great deterrent for overeating. During this second trimester of Albert's life, he always stayed trim, played tennis once a week, skied on weekends, and never failed to rest from his work one day per week.

When Albert was about 50, he noticed his knees beginning to ache when he came down the stairs in the morning. His doctor gave him a book on stretching exercises for the whole body. Albert began a new pursuit of wellness that day. In addition to his flexibility routine, he began doing 50 push-ups and 50 sit-ups each morning, followed by a 30-minute walk with his dog. To this day, 25 years later, you can still find Albert running through this routine—but not on Sundays.

When Jesus captured Albert's heart and devotion at the age of 36, his loyalty became evident. He has faithfully served the pastors and congregations of the churches he has attended. From his early beginning as a children's Sunday-school teacher to his later roles as building committee chairman, small-group leader, elder, and board member of a local youth-mentoring organization, Albert has kept active in his service for the kingdom.

At 75, Albert is still healthy, strong, and kingdom-minded. He continues to run his own company and is, in fact, considering starting another one. When asked what he thought about retirement he laughed and said, "I'm never going to retire!" Albert's life verse is Psalm 90:12, which I've heard him quote on a number of occasions: "Teach us to number our days aright, that we may gain a heart of wisdom." Let's take this verse to heart and be mindful that our days *are* numbered...

and that we can influence the number of days we live by gaining a heart of wisdom.

WHO SAYS I'M OLD?

A few years back I treated Joseph, a 90-year-old man who came to see me with the report of neck pain and stiffness. Prior to coming for physical therapy, he had been seen by his primary-care physician. Joseph had found his doctor to be less than sympathetic that day. His doctor had brusquely asked him, "What do you expect at ninety?" My patient, who was quite feisty, fired back, "I expect to feel like I did last week, when I *didn't* have neck pain!"

Good for you, sir! Six treatments later, and my patient wasn't only pain-free, he had 50 percent more rotation in his neck, making him a much safer driver. (Yes, Joseph still drove.) If a 90-year-old can act to improve his health, so can you. Without a doubt, better and lasting health is obtainable and maintainable. You simply need to make the effort to get involved in bringing it about. We have a job to do until the day we are called to our heavenly home. Let's be found *living* until the day we die. Amen?

Anna of Old

Shortly after Jesus' birth we find Mary and Joseph bringing Him to be dedicated at the temple. They are met by the third lifelong servant of the Lord I'd like you to consider. Anna, who was from the tribe of Asher, embodied her tribe's name, which when translated into English means to "*feel* blessed." Anna knew she was blessed as a daughter of the king, but she lived a life which demonstrated how she *felt*. In the Gospel of Luke we find this short description of her life:

> There was also a prophetess, Anna…She was very old…
> a widow until she was eighty-four. She never left the
> temple but worshiped night and day, fasting and praying.

> LUKE 2:36-37

Anna remained a vital pillar for her community by remaining active at the temple and by interceding with God on a daily basis. Scripture tells us that upon seeing Jesus in His mother's arms, she prophesies His future. I'm sure this wasn't the first encouraging prophecy this woman uttered. Likely she blessed many a frightened, directionless, and troubled soul in her days serving in the courts of the Lord. Let me introduce you to another such woman who continues, at the same age of Anna, to have an eternal impact on those she comes in contact with.

A Modern-Day Anna

Adeline Bruno was the child of Italian immigrants, born in the middle of the Roaring Twenties in Brooklyn, New York. Today she is 84 years young. Vibrant and full of energy, Adeline seems to have her hands in a lot these days. Every Tuesday morning you'll find her at church setting the tables and cutting the bagels for the women's Bible study. While the study is running, so is Adeline. She is downstairs in the nursery teaching the 3-to-5 year-olds! Sunday mornings during the first church service, you'll find her in the same location surrounded by bright-eyed toddlers. Weekday afternoons, Mrs. Bruno, the name by which she is better known, doesn't go home to rest. Rather she serves the community by teaching school-aged children how to sew, knit, and crochet at the local public elementary school's aftercare program.

Adeline, whose family was Catholic, began attending a Baptist church when she was 5 years old. At the age of 12, she asked Jesus to be her Savior while away at a Christian summer camp. Her service for the Lord, she says, comes in response to "just how good He has been to me my whole life. I am motivated by my love for Jesus and for the children."

Involvement in church and community isn't something new for this woman of 84. With her four young children in tow, Adeline helped convince her town of North Babylon, New York, to open its first public library. She recalls pulling a red wagon around her neighborhood to collect book donations for the shelves. In the church she's attended since 1964, Mrs. Bruno has assisted parents in raising their boys and girls with this amazing service record: Sunday-school teacher for 46 years and counting (she told the Sunday-school superintendent he could replace her when she turned 90!); Pioneer Girls leader for 14 years; vacation Bible school department head for 45 years; preschool teacher/director for 21 years.

Adeline has always tried to stay healthy by eating a diet heavy in fruits and vegetables, and low in starch. Forever a walker, she still walks 15 to 20 minutes two to three times a week (in good weather). Not giving a thought to her age, she returned to college at the age of 53 and earned an associate degree in early childhood education. When I asked Adeline what she thought about retirement, she said, "I never think about it. I just keep going. I love the children!" Her life verse is (not surprisingly) Philippians 4:13: "I can do all things through Christ who strengthens me" (NKJV).

● ● ●

In Romans 12:18 Paul gives this directive to the early church: "*As far as it depends on you,* live at peace with everyone." Paul knew that relationships would not always be peaceful, yet he still charged us to do our best with the part *we* had control over. Determine to have this same mind-set from today forward as you seek to restore and maintain your physical health. Even though we are not guaranteed a picture-perfect outcome, we must strive for a healthier tomorrow—as far as it depends on us. This way, in the end, no matter what the outcome, we can stand before God unashamed, knowing that we were faithful stewards of the health He gave us as His gift.

Throughout this book I have suggested many avenues for you to consider during your journey toward a healthier and more productive future. In closing this final chapter, I implore you—invest in your health today so you can gain a greater opportunity of enjoying every stage of your life in the future. You will never regret an investment in your wellness.

As the sun was setting on Moses' life, he spoke a prophecy over each of the 12 tribes of Israel. With his hand outstretched over the leader's head, he blessed the clan of Asher by declaring, "May your strength equal your days!" In effect, Moses was saying, "May you always be found healthy and strong—until the day God calls you home!" This day I join Moses in giving the same blessing to you. May *your* strength, my friend, match the number of *your* days—all for His glory, Amen! Hope to see you in heaven after a long and productive "run" down here.

Blessings to you,
Lisa

POINTS TO PONDER

1. What have my views of retirement been up to this point?

2. Have I set preconceived age limits on my acts of service and longevity of service within the church, my community, and around the world?

3. How will this teaching on the Bible's view of retirement impact my future?

4. What roles should I look to fill as I get into my sixties and beyond?

5. Who do I know who is where I want to be at their age?

6. When will I intentionally "interview" them so I can learn from their successes...and their mistakes?

7. What first step can I take today to ensure that "as far as it depends on me" my strength will equal my days?

Notes

Chapter 4—Rest for the Weary

1. J. Connor, R. Norton, S. Ameratunga, et al., "Driver sleepiness and risk of serious injury to car occupants: population based case control study," *BMJ* 324 (2002): 1125; Stephen Eller and Pamela Minkley, "The High Price of Sleep Deprivation," *RT for Decision Makers in Respiratory Care,* June/July 1998.

2. J.M. Ellenbogen, "Cognitive benefits of sleep and their loss due to sleep deprivation," *Neurology* 64 (2005 Apr 12): E25-7.

3. R.C. Kessler, W.T. Chiu, O. Demler, and E.E. Walters, "Prevalence, severity, and comorbidity of twelve-month DSM-IV disorders in the National Comorbidity Survey Replication (NCS-R)," *Archives of General Psychiatry* 62 (2005 Jun): 617-27.

4. M. Irwin, M. McClintick, J. Costlow, C. Fortner, M. White, J.C. Gillin, "Partial night sleep deprivation reduces natural killer and cellular immune responses in humans," *FASEB Journal* 10, no. 5 (1996): 643-653.

5. K. Spiegel, K. Knutson, R. Leproult, E. Tasali, E. Van Cauter, "Sleep loss: a novel risk factor for insulin resistance and Type 2 diabetes," *J Applied Physiology* 99, no. 5 (2005 Nov): 2008-19.

Chapter 5—Fueling Up for the Road Ahead

1. S.T. St. Jeor, B.V. Howard, T.E. Prewitt, V. Bovee, T. Bazzarre, R.H. Eckel, "Dietary protein and weight reduction: a statement for healthcare professionals from the Nutrition Committee of the Council on Nutrition, Physical Activity, and Metabolism of the American Heart Association," *Circulation* 104 (2001): 1869-1874.

2. St. Jeor et al.

3. J. Balch and P. Balch, *Prescription for Nutritional Healing* (New York: Avery Publishing Group, 1998), 12-20.

4. Vaughns One-Page Summaries, "Vitamin-Mineral chart," www.vaughns-1-pagers.com/food/vitamin-mineral-chart.htm, accessed 2010 Jan 7.

5. National Cancer Institute, "Antioxidants and Cancer Prevention: Fact Sheet," www.cancer.gov/cancertopics/factsheet/prevention/antioxidants, accessed 2010 Jan 7.

6. Arthur Agatston, *The South Beach Diet Supercharged* (New York: Rodale, Inc, 2008), 84.

7. M.W. Gillman et al., "Protective Effect of Fruits and Vegetables on Development of Stroke in Men," *Journal of the American Medical Association* 273 (1995): 1113; J.M. Gaziano et al., "A prospective study of consumption of carotenoids in fruits and vegetables and decreased cardiovascular mortality in the elderly," *Annals of Epidemiology* 5 (1995): 255-260; G.A. Colditz et al., "Increased green and yellow vegetable intake and lowered cancer deaths in an elderly

population," *American Journal of Clinical Nutrition* 41 (1985): 32; E. Giovannucci et al., "A Prospective Study of Tomato Products, Lycopene, and Prostate Cancer Risk," *Journal of the National Cancer Institute* 87 (1995): 1767; J.M. Seddon et al., "Dietary Carotenoids, Vitamins A, C, and E, and Advanced Age-Related Macular Degeneration," *Journal of the American Medical Association* 272 (1994): 1413.

8. C.M. Albert et al., "Fish consumption and risk of sudden cardiac death," *Journal of the American Medical Association* 279 (1998): 23.

9. Ernest B. Hawkins and Steven D. Ehrlich. "Omega-3 Fatty Acids," University of Maryland Medical Center, www.umm.edu/altmed/articles/omega-3-000316.htm, accessed 2010 Jan 13.

10. Mayo Clinic Staff, "Dietary Fiber: Essential for a healthy body," www.mayoclinic.com/health/fiber, accessed 2010 Jan 13.

11. Mayo Clinic Staff, "High fiber foods," November 17, 2009, www.mayoclinic.com/health/high-fiber-foods, accessed 2010 Jan 14.

12. R. Huxley et al., "Coffee, Decaffeinated Coffee, and Tea Consumption in Relation to Incident Type 2 Diabetes Mellitus: A Systematic Review with Meta-analysis," *Arch Intern Med* 169, no. 22 (2009): 2053-2063.

13. I.-H. Lin et al., "Smoking, green tea consumption, genetic polymorphisms in the insulin-like growth factors and lung cancer risk," *AACR-IASLC* 2010; abstract A21.

Chapter 6—Waist Not, Want Not

1. Craig Freudenrich, "How Fat Cells Work," http://health.howstuffworks.com/fat-cell.htm, accessed 2010 Jan 25.

2. Johns Hopkins Bloomberg School of Public Health, "Waist Size Linked to Diabetes Risk in Adult Men," *ScienceDaily,* 28 March 2005, www.sciencedaily.com/releases/2005/03/050325150149.htm, accessed 16 September 2009.

3. University of California—Los Angeles. "Waist-hip Ratio Better Than BMI for Gauging Obesity in Elderly, Study Finds," *ScienceDaily,* 2 September 2009, www.sciencedaily.com/releases/2009/09/090901150951.htm, accessed 16 September 2009.

4. Cheryle Hart and Mary Kay Grossman, *The Insulin-Resistance Diet* (New York: McGraw Hill, 2008), 31-34.

5. Arthur Agatston, *The South Beach Diet Supercharged* (New York: Rodale, Inc, 2008), 13.

6. Lisa Morrone, *Overcoming Overeating* (Eugene, OR: Harvest House Publishers, 2009), 167-168.

7. Positive Health Steps, "Calories burned per activity chart," October 5, 2009, http://positivehealthsteps.com/calories-burned.shtml, accessed 2010 February 25.

Chapter 8—The 10-Minute Muscle Makeover

1. F. Martini, *Anatomy and Physiology,* 5th ed., chap. 10: "Muscle Tissue" (Upper Saddle River, NJ: Prentice-Hall, 2005), http://cwx.prenhall.com/bookbind/pubbooks/martinidemo/chapter10/medialib/CH10/html/ch10_5_3.html.

Chapter 9—Put the Brakes on Brain Aging

1. Mayo Clinic Staff, "Dementia," April 17, 2009, www.mayoclinic.com/health/dementia/DS01131/DSECTION=symptoms, accessed 2010 March 16.

2. Daniel Amen, *Making a Good Brain Great* (New York: Crown Publishing Group, 2005), 86.

3. Institute for Natural Resources (INR), "Brain Aging After 30" seminar, 2007.

4. J.P. Nilsson et al., "Less effective executive function after one night's sleep deprivation," *J Sleep Research* 14, no. 1 (2005 Mar): 1-6.

5. Paul E. Bendheim, *The Brain Training Revolution.* (Naperville, IL: Source Books, 2009), 256-257.

6. Cynthia Green and the editors of *Prevention* magazine, *Brain Power Game Plan* (New York: Rodale, Inc., 2009), 50.

7. Green, 56.

8. Green, 12.

9. Green, 44.

10. Green, 11.

11. Green, 68.

12. Green, 68.

13. Bendheim, 56.

14. Bendheim, 239-240.

15. Amen, 180.

Chapter 10—Retirement—Moses' Style

1. "The History of Retirement, from Early Man to A.A.R.P.," *New York Times,* March 20, 1999, www.nytimes.com/1999/03/21/jobs/the-history-of-retirement-from-early-man-to-aarp.html, accessed 2010 April 12.

This day…I have set before you life
and death, blessings and curses.
Now choose life, so that you and your children
may live and that you may love the LORD your
God, listen to his voice, and hold fast to him.
For the LORD is your life,
and he will give you many years…

DEUTERONOMY 30:19-20

Lisa Morrone graduated magna cum laude from the Physical Therapy program at the State University of New York at Stony Brook in 1989, receiving a bachelor of science degree in physical therapy. In addition to her college education, Lisa has taken over 30 continuing education courses in the area of orthopedic physical therapy. As a physical therapist, Lisa has been treating patients in the field of orthopedic rehabilitation for over two decades now. In 1990 she accepted the position of adjunct professor at Touro College, Bay Shore, New York, which she still holds today.

At Touro College Lisa instructs in the Doctorate Program in Physical Therapy. Presently Lisa co-teaches Musculoskeletal II (Spinal Orthopedics) and an advanced elective on Spinal Muscle Energy Techniques (evaluation and treatment specific to the spinal joints). Her past teaching credits also include Massage, Extremity Joint Mobilization (evaluation and treatment of the joints in the arms and legs), Spinal Stabilization Training (core strengthening of the trunk, hips, and shoulder-blade muscles), and Kinesiology (the study of bones, muscles, and joints and their roles in the human body).

Lisa's library of self-help health books began with *Overcoming Back and Neck Pain*, published in February 2007. Lisa is a graduate of both the speaker and the writer tracks of the She Speaks Conference (Proverbs 31 Ministries), where she was assessed at the highest level of proficiency. As a speaker, Lisa has taught in both secular (community and medical) and church-based settings. Lisa makes her home on Long Island, New York, along with her husband, daughter, and son.

Restoring Your Temple™

Within Christian circles, one's physical body is often referred to as the temple of the Holy Spirit. The reason for this is found in 1 Corinthians 6:19, where the Bible says, "Do you not know that your body is the temple of the Holy Spirit, who is in you, whom you received from God?" Temples are places where worship takes place. But what exactly is worship? To quote author Rick Warren

> Worship is far more than praising, singing, and praying to God. Worship is a lifestyle of *enjoying* God, *loving* him and *giving* ourselves to be used for his purposes. When you use your life for God's glory, everything you do can become an act of worship.

Romans 12:1 further tells us to "offer your *bodies* as living sacrifices, holy and pleasing to God—this is your spiritual act of worship." God has plans for your body...physical plans. Your hands and feet are meant to be used as his hands and feet on this earth. So whether He calls you to raise children, teach Sunday school, or work with teenagers or the homeless, you need a physical body that is ready for action. Scripture says: "The harvest is plentiful, but the workers are few." Often this is because the workers are at doctor's appointments, are going to physical therapy, or are simply so tired they can't get off the couch!

It is the intent of **Restoring Your Temple** to enable the Body of Christ to perform the work of Christ. The longer you live in good physical health, the greater your capacity to serve God will be, and the more you will be able to enjoy the abundant life God has promised to his children.

Visit Lisa Morrone's website, **www.LisaMorrone.com,** for free resources that include

- a BMI (body mass index) calculator
- a home exercise program for those suffering with jaw pain (TMD)
- downloadable headache tracking charts
- guidance on how to find a good physical therapist
- a source of "Lisa-tested," quality health-related products
- quick tips for back, neck, head, or jaw pain and blood-sugar regulation
- helpful articles on health-related issues
- the complete library of Lisa's books, including *Overcoming Headaches and Migraines*

More Life-Changing Help from Lisa Morrone
and Harvest House Publishers

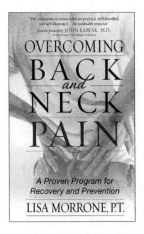

Overcoming Back and Neck Pain
A Proven Program for Recovery and Prevention

From 20 years of teaching and practicing physical therapy, Lisa Morrone gives you a way to say *no* to the treadmill of prescriptions, endless treatments, and a limited lifestyle. This straightforward, clinically proven approach shows you how to…

- benefit from good posture and "core stability"
- strengthen and stretch key muscles
- shift to healthy movement patterns
- recover from pain caused by compressed or degenerated discs
- address "inside issues" that affect healing—nutrition, rest, and emotional/spiritual struggles

"The treatments Lisa recommends are practical, well described, and well illustrated…An invaluable resource."

JOHN LABIAK, MD, ORTHOPAEDIST AND SPINAL SURGEON

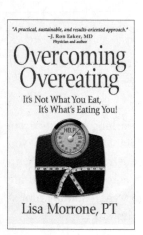

"A practical, sustainable, and results-oriented approach."
–J. Ron Eaker, MD
Physician and author

Overcoming Overeating
It's Not What You Eat,
It's What's Eating You!

Lisa Morrone, PT

Overcoming Overeating
It's Not What You Eat, It's What's Eating You!

Health author Lisa Morrone bypasses diet plans and zeros in on *heart* plans—because food isn't typically the real problem. Here are tools to assess *yourself* (not just your food intake), followed by tested methods for breaking through the food trap from the inside out. You'll find ways to

- identify and address the underlying causes of your overeating

- avoid using food as a time-filler, mood elevator, or painkiller

- find freedom to achieve steady, solid results from any reputable weight-loss method

- *finally* keep the weight off, feel better about yourself, and improve your overall health

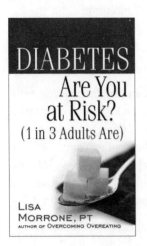

Diabetes

Are You at Risk? (1 in 3 Adults Are)

You could be one of the 60 million American adults with prediabetes. Why? Because most people with this condition *don't know they have it.* And an additional 7 million adults don't know they have full-blown diabetes!

Diabetes: Are You at Risk? will help you find out where *you* stand. Better yet, it will show you how to stop or even reverse the consequences of untreated blood-sugar problems. This can-do, action-oriented resource points the way toward a longer, healthier, more productive life—a life that will benefit you and those close to you.

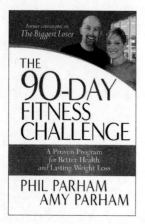

The 90-Day Fitness Challenge
A Proven Program for Better Health and Lasting Weight Loss

Phil and Amy Parham

You've tried the diet plans with little success. Now let Phil and Amy Parham, former contestants on NBC's *The Biggest Loser,* show you how to transform your life and live your dreams of being healthier, happier, and more fit. *The 90-Day Fitness Challenge* is a faith-based, informative, and motivational book that will

- take you step-by-step through a 90-day program for permanent weight loss
- provide you simple and practical healthy food and fitness plans
- point the way toward developing better eating habits and an active lifestyle
- incorporate Scripture and faith principles to encourage you to make God a part of your journey

The Parhams know from experience the obstacles to fitness that you face. Allow them to come alongside to inspire, motivate, and provide practical life skills on your 90-day journey toward better health and lasting weight loss.